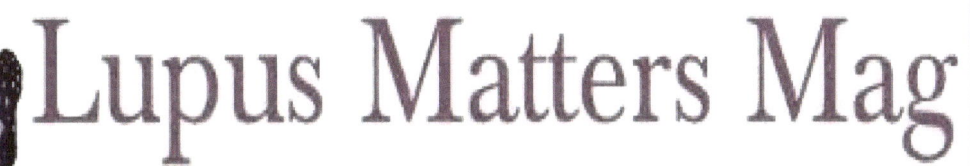

Lupus Matters Mag

Lupus Matters Corporation

SPRING 2017

Contents

Stage Play info
Lupus Matters Cover Contest
LMC Facebook Page

from the FOUNDER

We are excited about this PREMIER issue of the Lupus Matters Magazine. It's the first of many to come.

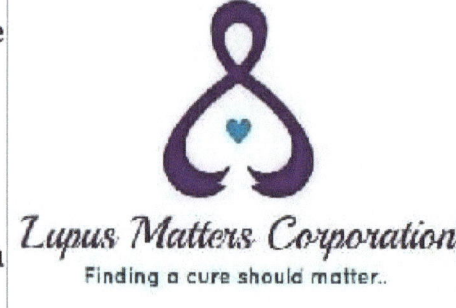

Lupus Matters Corporation
Finding a cure should matter..

Hi this is Monica, CEO of Lupus Matters Corporation. At our Corporation we pride ourselves on the education and awareness of Lupus.

Our main goal is to provide an uplifting Atmosphere by encouraging and supporting those with this ugly disease to live life to the fullest. In order to live better we have to think better. Better about eating, exercising and our daily activities. We also wants to provide you with substantial information and articles, for success with lupus.

So join the movement and hashtag #lupusmatters on social media.

For more information call 404-997-0761 or simply log onto www.lupusmatters.org

To become a sponsor, volunteer or to donate funds, email us at lupusmatters@gmail.com

Finally Lupus Matters Corporation would like to thank everyone for their support.

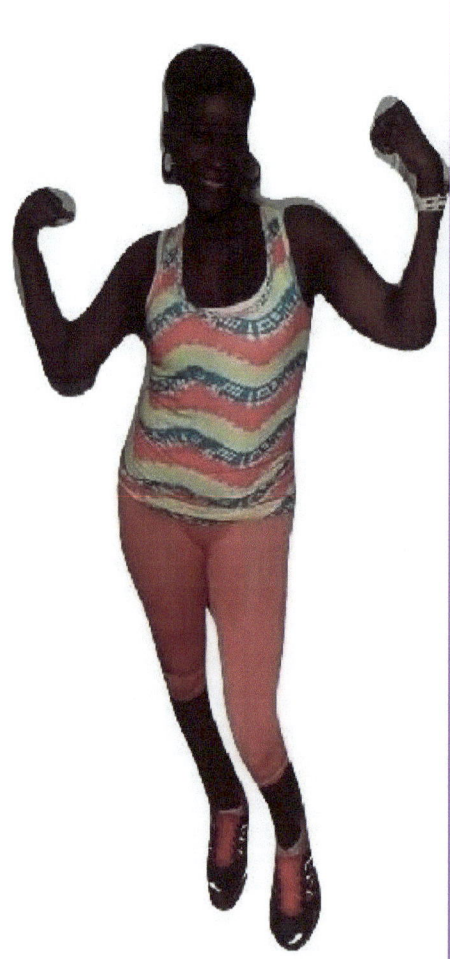

Warm Regards,

Monica Ellis

LET OUR PEOPLE

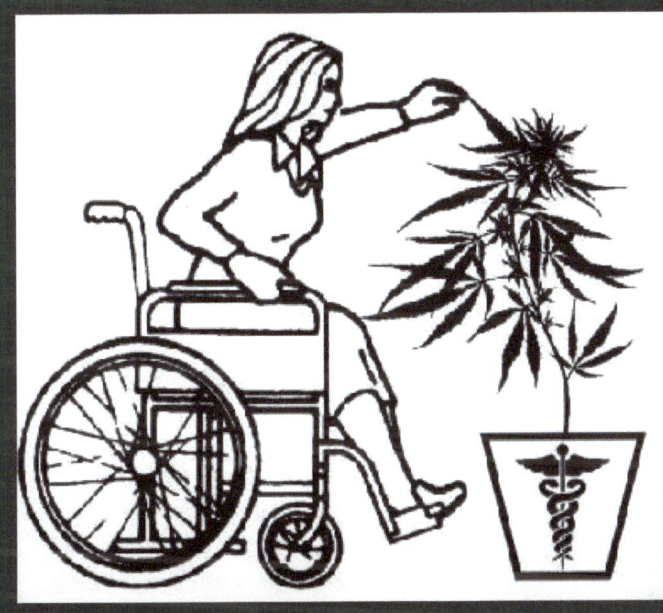

GROW

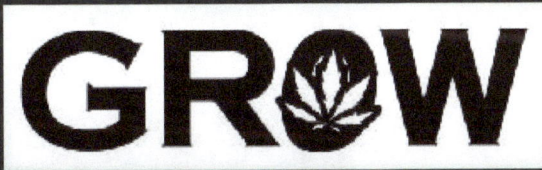

THE MARIJUANA SAGA CONTINUES

By

BRIDGET DANDARAW-SERITT

Healing the world through:

- Education
- Community Improvement
- Ending Stigma

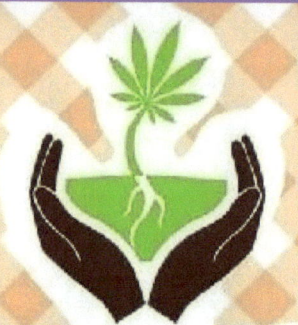

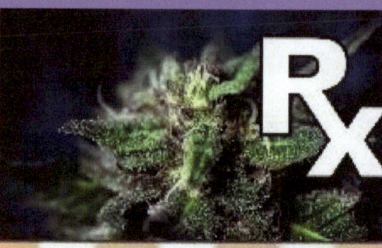

LEGALIZE

CANNA-PATIENT
RESOURCE CONNECTION

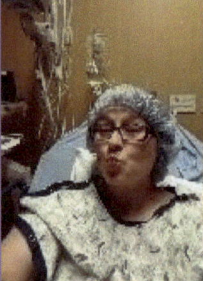

About Bridget

My family is absolutely amazing. Harlin and I have 3 children combined, 2 incredible daughters and a fabulous son! I also have an amazing Granddaughter! I love my life and am so blessed to have an incredible husband who has shown unconditional love for me. Meeting the "one" and blending my family has been a wild adventure and I look forward to every day I have with them!

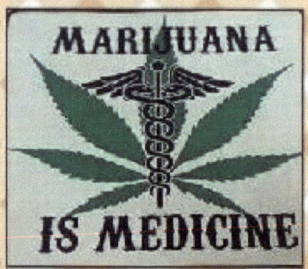

MARIJUANA IS MEDICINE

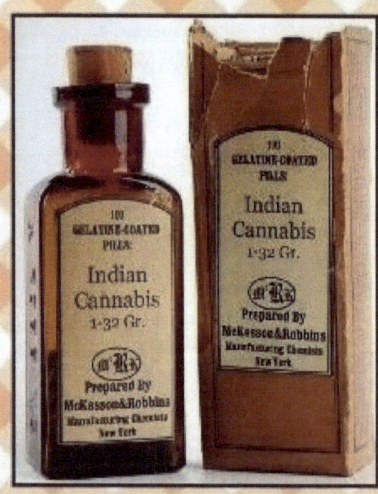

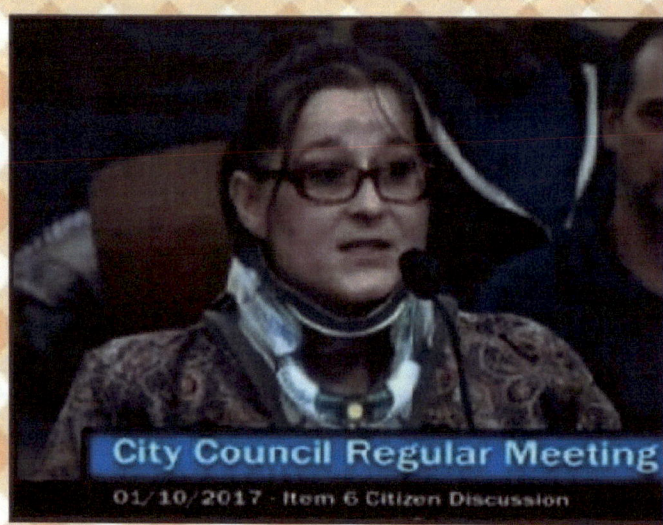

City Council Regular Meeting
01/10/2017 · Item 6 Citizen Discussion

Legalizing Cannabis would help Chronic Pain sufferers.

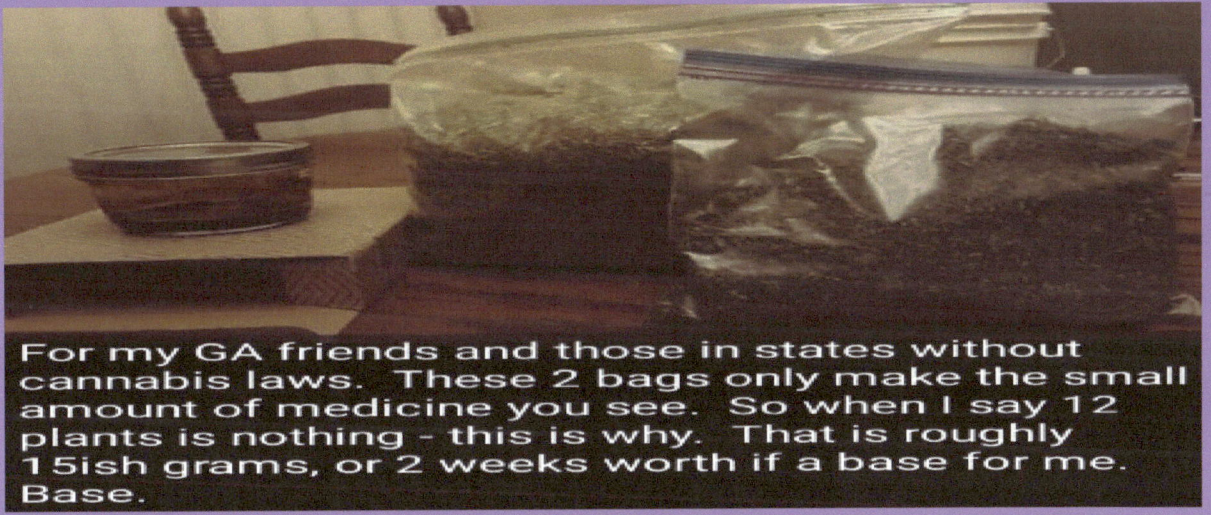

For my GA friends and those in states without cannabis laws. These 2 bags only make the small amount of medicine you see. So when I say 12 plants is nothing - this is why. That is roughly 15ish grams, or 2 weeks worth if a base for me. Base.

Advice to a newly diagnosed Lupie? I know lupus is a scary diagnosis, but my advice is to connect with other patients, educate yourself, and let go of your views on "imperfections". Connecting with other patients is essential. My husband said it best when he told me, "You can only relate to what you have experienced. Since the worst pain most people experience is a stubbed toe, in their eyes - you have a stubbed toe." The patient community understands your frustrations and can even offer coping suggestions. As alone as we feel, connecting with the patient community can show you just how "normal" in this you are. Educating yourself is key. Now that you have been diagnosed with lupus, very well-meaning friends will start coming out of the wood work with "cures" and remedies their friends tried. While many of those have the possibility of easing symptoms, there is no cure. Know you will have to do what works for you, and that these diseases present differently in everyone. What works for one, may not work for you and vice versa. Know what lupus is and how it works, so you can choose the best treatment path for you. Lastly, let go of any negative thoughts and excessive perfectionist standards. These will only cause depression and most of these are unrealistic. One of the most voiced wishes is "I just want to be like I was before." Unfortunately, that almost never happens, and ignoring how to live with your disease in hopes of magically curing it, often causes severe depression. Learn how to enjoy life and live with your disease. This way, you are even happier if you end up being one of the ones that goes into a permanent remission!

http://gangaautoimmuner.blogwritr.com/2014/06/25/life-lesson-2-be-okay-with-imperfections/

http://gangaautoimmuner.blogwritr.com/2014/05/20/autoimmuner-life-lessons-1-be-a-stubborn-horses-arse/

Toughest challenges? Symptom wise, fatigue is my toughest challenge. It is like having all my muscles injected with lead. It takes my body 10 times as much energy to perform a task as it normally does, and during fatigue flares it is difficult to do anything. Fatigue is not being tired, but having no physical ability to do even the most menial tasks.

Mentally, I think my biggest challenge is asking for help. Often, we tend to feel like burdens when we ask for help, and I am no different. I hate admitting that something is too much for me to handle or that I need assistance. On flare days, I don't contribute much to my family's chore routine and that causes the most horrible guilt. I am very lucky and have a family that understands, but I still struggle with asking for help and those feeling of guilt.

What would I teach a total stranger?   This is a very difficult question for me. There are so many things I would want a stranger to know about life with lupus and autoimmune diseases. From explaining how lupus symptoms change from day to day, to how there are very few medications that help the disease, to how those with lupus often end up with other co-morbidities - all of these are essential things to know. However, I think I would teach a total stranger compassion - not just for lupus or even those who are sick, but to show compassion to all other beings on this planet. Compassion is the key to finding cures, to functioning in society, and the key to a better and inclusive future for all. This concept applies to all humans from the homeless man on the corner, to the mentally ill addict that needs compassionate help. So, I can firmly say that I would teach compassion when talking to strangers.

How do I enjoy life? Thanks to my children, I could teach myself how to enjoy life. As a parent, you are responsible for supplementing their education and teaching them how to be adults. A child tends to find joy in the simplest of things. The falling leaves of Autumn, butterflies on a flower, sunsets over the mountains, and smiles in humans all carry the potential to lift us up each day - if we allow it. I spent several years training myself to find something beautiful in as many situations as possible. Now it is an automatic thing, and I don't notice all the bad stuff as much. I am still horribly sick, still in pain every single day, and still have bad things happen. That has not changed, and it never changes for anyone. This is life. However, this life experience is what we make of it. I plan to make this the best Autoimmune Life ever! http://gangaautoimmuner.blogwritr.com/2015/05/06/life-is-too-short-for-dry-socks/

What alternative treatments would I recommend? This is highly individual as autoimmune disease presents differently in every person. Diet plays a crucial role in how severe symptoms can get, and our food is fuel. I would recommend an elimination diet and designing your own customized plan. Be sure you add those foods that fight inflammation and avoid those that create it! Not everyone has the same sensitivities, so keep a food journal!

I personally have found amazing relief using Phyto cannabinoid therapy. Medical marijuana has replaced my DMARD (methotrexate), steroids, opiates, sleeping aids, Plaquenil, nerve agents (anti-seizure drugs for neuropathy), NSAIDS, and more. When I have access to proper medical marijuana dosing, my diseases tend to go into remission or at least hit the "mild" activity level.   Marijuana use has shown significant promise for 3 main disease categories, as well as hope for many others. The three main families seeing great results from Phyto cannabinoid therapy are:

Cancers/Leukemia's, seizure disorders, and autoimmune diseases. If this is something you have access to, I would highly recommend taking advantage of your state's program!

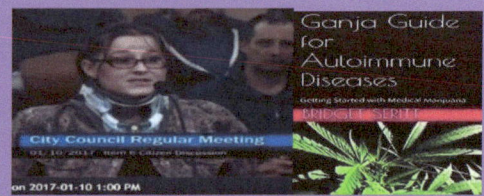

To learn more about this movement, help end the stigma against patients and to protect the rights of patients.

Like "**Canna-Patient Resource Connection**" on Facebook

Medical Marijuana & Lupus

Cannabis is considered an ideal medication to help Lupus patients cope with the symptoms of the disorder like nausea and pain. It's also known to be an anti-inflammatory, suppressing certain parts of the immune system.

"These endocannabinoids are serious contenders to try and alleviate pain and inflammation in rheumatic diseases. We need to stop sniggering about it and talk about it, and embrace them with the necessary caution of course."

Rheumatology Expert: Medical Marijuana Needs Serious Consideration

(Photo: the New Project)

A rheumatology expert from Dalhousie University believes medical marijuana could be very useful for managing pain and inflammation in arthritis, but needs to be taken more seriously by those in the field.

Dr. McDougall has conducted research on the use of cannabinoids and endocannabinoids in treating osteoarthritis. In an earlier talk on "The Basic Science of Chronic Pain," he noted that 36% of authorized marijuana patients in Canada were smoking marijuana to treat arthritis.

Moving Beyond~ God won't give you more than you can handle...

I am 36 years and the mother of two children, a 16-year-old son and 11-year-old daughter. I was recently diagnosed with an autoimmune disease called LUPUS in 2014. I started out with just having chest pains bad; I was in and out of the ER twice a week. I either came by ambulance or a family member took me. The last episode I was at work November 2014 and I was having bad chest pains. My coworkers rushed me to the ER, by the time they got me there I was hyperventilating. I started having chest pains in March of 2014 so as you can see 8 months I was in and out of the ER and doctor's office and no one knew what was going on with me. I even saw a chronic pain management doctor did steroid injections in my chest to help with the pain. The second to last time I was in the ER they said I had something called Costochondritis which is inflammation of the breast bone. They sent me home with pain medication and said follow up with your primary care doctor. I did this and I wasn't getting any relief they said I needed to see a rheumatoid doctor to get a better look at the inside of my body. I went through an intensive study at George Washington hospital in Washington, DC rheumatoid team. The next step they said that I would have to have Benlysta infusions well the first three would be every two weeks and then once every 4 weeks. I was scared and had no clue as to why they wanted to give me this medication when they haven't explained to me what was going on.

I had to stop working. That last visit to the ER in November was the last day I stepped foot at my job that I had over 15 years of experience in. I was admitted in November 2014 with fluid around my heart which is called parricidal infusion. I also my right lung was collapsed onto top pneumonia. I was taken to the room where I thought I would get the care I needed for a few days and go home. Well I was there for 3 days just when they were going to send me home I took the turn for the worst. They had me up and walking around, well the day I was to get up I couldn't walk my feet were shuffling and making it hard to take a step. The same day I was eating my lunch and my mom said why are you shaking your hands, I said "I'm not shaking "I look down and I was indeed shaking. They had to call the rehabilitation doctor to come and evaluate you. He told them that I had tremors, but he was stumped as to what was going on with me; he told the nurses that I needed to be switched over to his department. My couple day stay turned into weeks in the rehabilitation unit of the Hospital. I had the infectious disease doctors from Georgetown University to come over and evaluate me. They were stumped as to why I could walk. My inflammation marker was sky high. While in the rehabilitation unit I had a speech, physical and occupational therapist to help me with my tremors. At 34, my whole world came crashing down on me with no warning signs. I couldn't even look at myself in the mirror. I cried 24/7 my look had changed because I was on some many medications. I was on prednisone 85 mg a day that I developed what we call the "**moon face**".

I never thought in a million years that I would be going through such devastation. Unable to walk on my own, my daughter embarrassed & didn't want me to come to her school, not wanting the kids to make fun of her. Although it hurt my heart, I took a backseat until I could walk with my cane. I spoke with my daughter to let her know that she didn't have to worry about what people think of me. God is in control and we all must have faith.

When I changed health insurance and found a new doctor. I went from thirty-five pills a day, down to seven pills a day. Being diagnosed with LUPUS, RA, Peripheral Neuropathy and partial retinal detachment felt like a death sentence... But with my new health team, we have found a regimen that is keeping me labs steady and my markers down. I do have minor setbacks. But, in my journey dealing with LUPUS, I came across a friend whom I find very dear to my heart. She sent me a CD that she made and it helps me when I'm going through a flare up. Song is called "Ta All My LUPIE Chix" Lupus Anthem. Lupus really does matter and we need to find a cure. Lupus is autoimmune disease that does not run in my family and we are still puzzled as to how I have it. People say you don't look sick. Just Lupus is unseen on the outside doesn't mean a person is not going through hell and high water on the inside.

I cry to myself because the pain is unbearable live with at times. Lupus is not an easy pill to swallow, I was in denial and scared because I have two beautiful kids looking up to me. It hurt me to my core to see the pain in my kid's eyes when I was having a flare up and they had to call 911 to get mommy help. With the grace of God, we made it through some difficult times.

People say to me Charlissa, you went through this storm and it made you stronger, I didn't think so at the time. Now I say that God wouldn't put anything on me that he knows that I can't handle.

I NEVER imagined that my life would get back to normal but Slowly in 2015, I came off the heavy steroids and start shedding all that weight from the medications. I started getting out more; letting people know that LUPUS is not contagious and that I am living my life to the fullest.

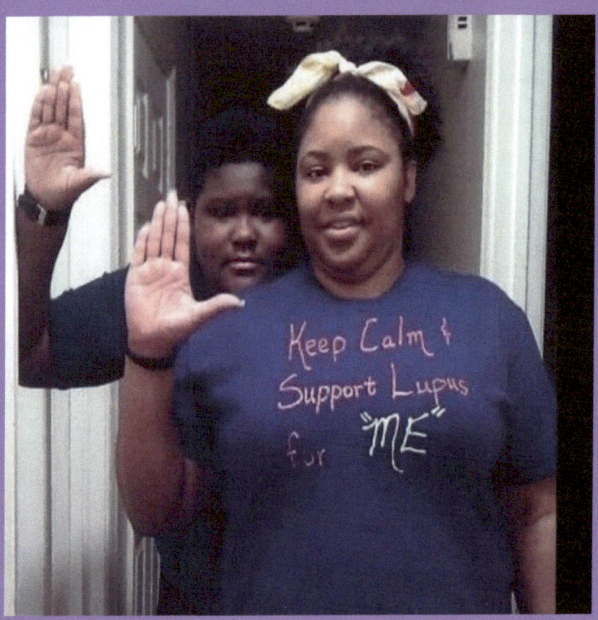 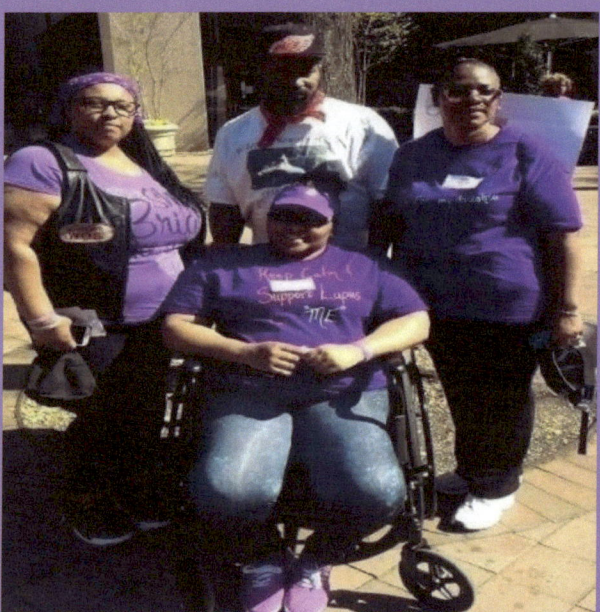

Clothing Donations Needed!!

Items Needed
- Uniform Tops
- Uniform Bottoms
- Socks
- Shoes
- Jackets

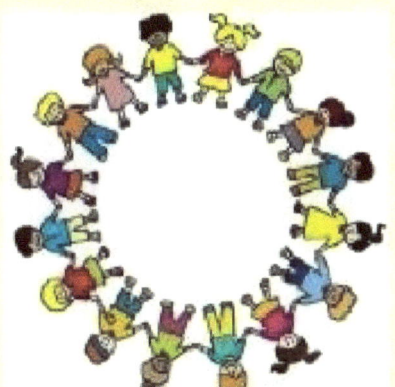

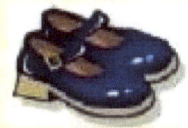

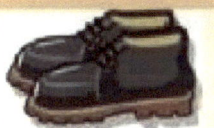

Clothing for a CURE!!!

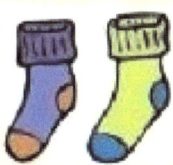

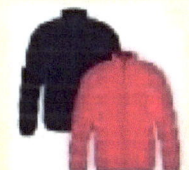

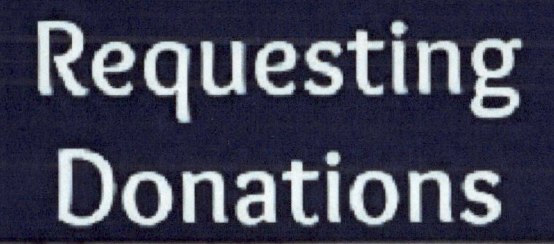

Requesting Donations

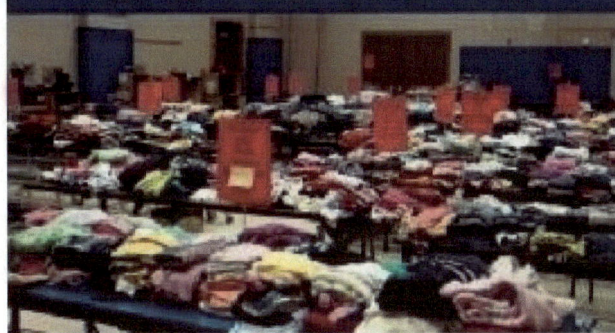

Lupus Matters Corporation

Finding a cure should matter..

Your donation is greatly appreciated

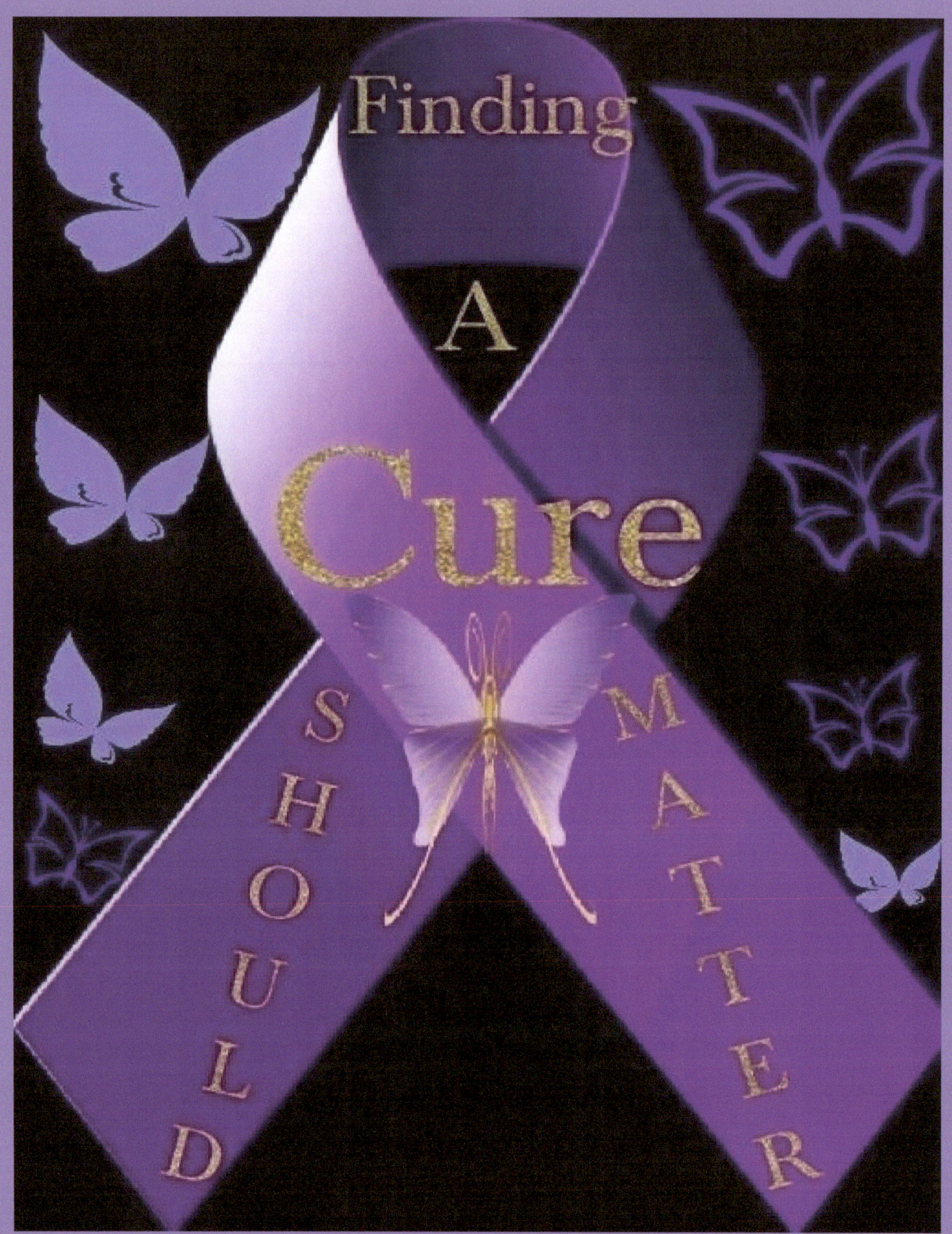

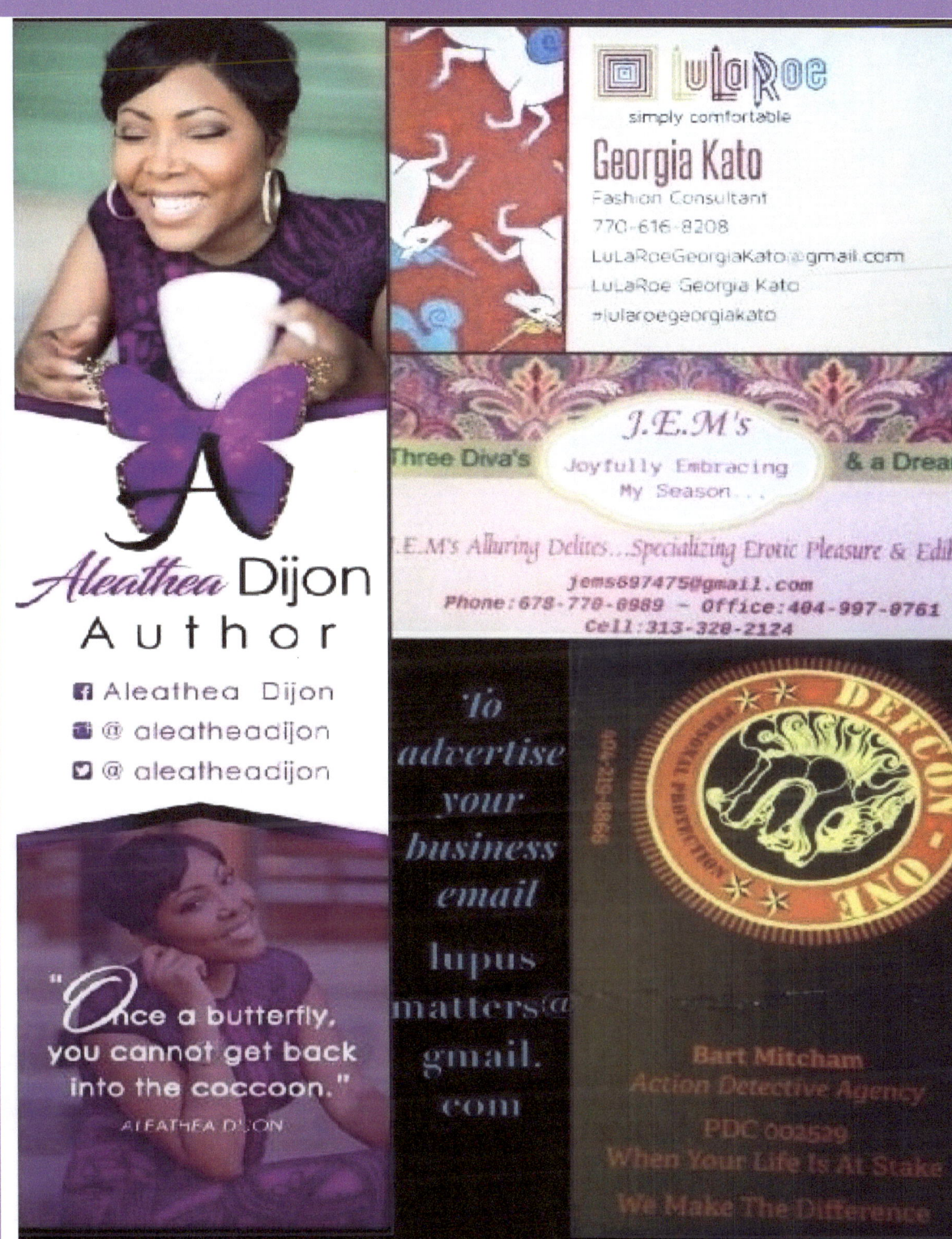

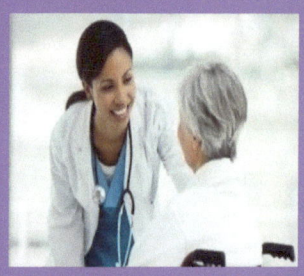

Key questions

TO ASK YOUR DOCTOR

REVIEW WITH YOUR DOCTOR TODAY!

Fill out this worksheet and review with your Rheumatologist.

1. How do you determine if my LUPUS is mild, moderate or severe?
   _____

2. How do you determine if my LUPUS is getting worse?
   _____

3. Are there any test to determine the severity of my illness?
   _____

4. Based on my symptoms and test results what medication(s) do you recommend?
   _____

5. What are the latest treatment options, and would any of them be right for me?
   _____

6. What types of exercise are safe for me to do? What other lifestyle changes do you recommend?
   _____

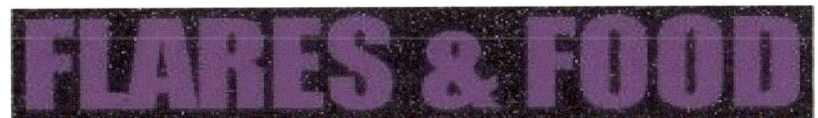

FLARES & FOOD

What Are You Doing?

Did you know the average American diet is loaded with sugar? Almost everything you see in a major grocery store, including the genetically altered vegetables, has unnecessary sugar in them. Sugar is a catalyst for many of the **diseases** that we see today. These diseases include, and are not limited to, diabetes, obesity, heart disease, and even cancer. WARNING: SUGAR IS ADDICTED

In a standard sized sugar cube, there are about 2.3 grams of sugar, while the recommended total daily limit for an individual intake is about 24 grams of sugar. This is one drink out of an entire day of eating and drinking many other things. Do you see where this conversation is going? Hey, try this! Next time you are craving your favorite soft drink or canned juice, check the back label for its ingredients. To find out how much sugar is in that product, multiply the serving amount by the grams of sugar per serving (i.e. 2.5 servings per can x 25 grams serving = 62.5 grams of sugar). Yikes, check it out! Even if you cut that in half (12 gram sugar limit intake daily), your body would still be getting more than enough sugar! We really do not need **any processed sugar to survive at ALL.**

If your body is unhealthy, combating ailments, or overloaded with sugary toxins, hit the gym or the steam room. Drink lots of water and sweat, sweat, sweat! Weight loss is another great way to regain control of your body's health. Fat pockets on the body carry many toxins that, if not moved, can lead to very serious diseases, even death. So, let us explore some more proactive choices that one can make to improve their overall health.

Things you can do:
- Move toward a "processed" sugar free diet (i.e. no soft drinks, gas station treats, cookies, cakes, and more)
- Replace "processed" sugar with natural fruit sugars
- COOK YOUR OWN FOOD (many times this is overlooked)
- Develop a habit of working out (**THIS IS KEY for removing toxins**)
- Eat all natural foods from the local farmer's market near you (organic and all natural are different)
- Integrate alkaline water into your normal drinking water
- Kale with every meal (the benefits are unreal)
- Remove fatty, sugary, foods from your house COMPLETELY (it will take time but it is possible)
- Bring homemade lunch and snacks to work
- Find out your blood type and **EAT TO YOUR BLOOD TYPE**

Ultimately, what you put in your body determines what your body can and cannot do. A healthy body and a healthy mind really go hand in hand. Therefore, the final question that you should be asking yourself NOW is (drum roll please)...

What are you doing and what are you going to do for yourself? The power to change and improve yourself... begins with YOU!

Karla Thomas

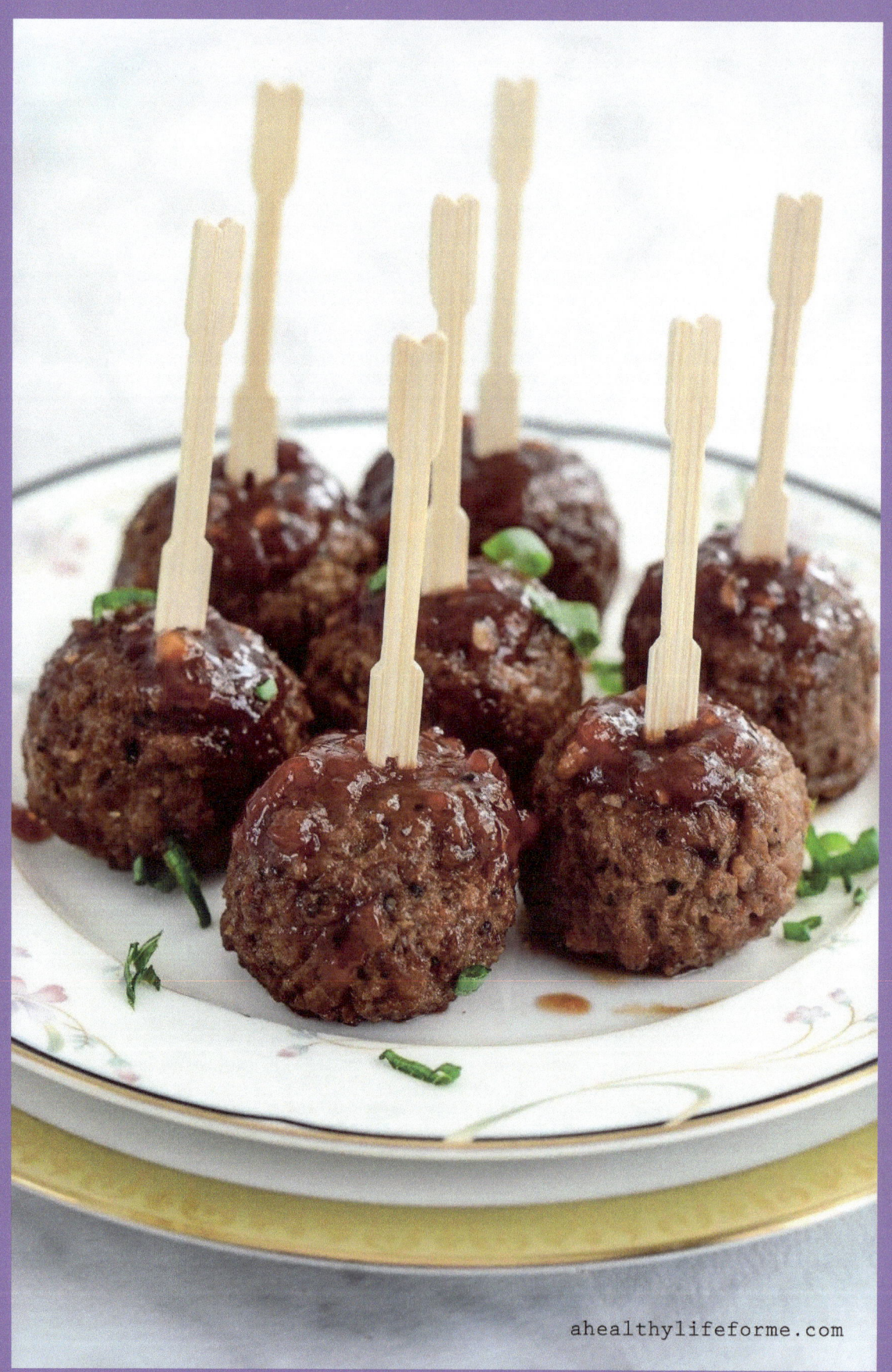

ahealthylifeforme.com

INGREDIENTS

- 1 package of Gardein Classic Meatless Meatballs {12 meatballs}

Sauce:
- ½ cup ketchup
- ½ cup maple syrup
  Coupons
- 2 tablespoons water
- 1-1/2 tablespoons apple cider vinegar
- 2 teaspoons Worcestershire sauce
- 1 tablespoon finely grated shallot, from one shallot
- 1 small clove garlic, minced
- ⅛ teaspoon ground black pepper
- ½ teaspoon salt

Toppings:
- 1 green onion, green parts only, diced

INSTRUCTIONS

Sauce:
1. Combine all the ingredients in a small bowl and whisk to blend.
2. Set a large skillet over medium heat and add sauce and Gardein Classic Meatless Meatballs.
3. Cover and cook till meatballs are heated through center, about 13-15 minutes.
4. Remove from heat, plate and top with remaining sauce from pan and sprinkle green onion.
5. Serve and Enjoy

VEGAN PROTEINS

PLANTS PROVIDE ALL OF THE ESSENTIAL AMINO ACIDS AND LOWER YOUR RISK OF HEART DISEASE AND CANCER (UNLIKE MEAT WHICH PROMOTES BOTH HEART DISEASE AND CANCER)

Note: Combining proteins in a single meal to form 'complete proteins' is based on outdated science and is unnecessary. If you're meeting your recommended calorie intake it's extremely likely you will also be consuming all the amino acids in sufficient quantities during the day. On average vegans actually obtain *70% more protein than required* per day -- there is no shortage of protein on a plant-based diet!

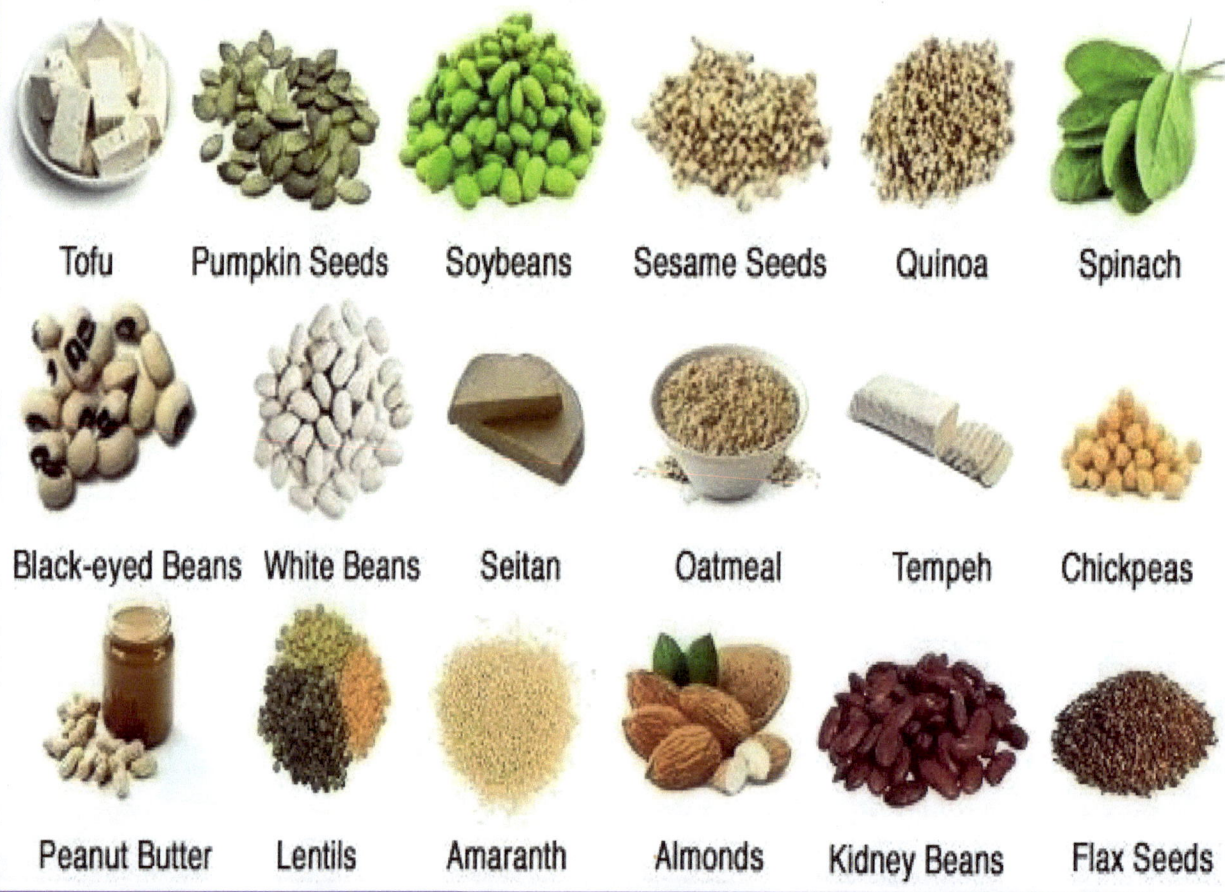

Tofu	Pumpkin Seeds	Soybeans	Sesame Seeds	Quinoa	Spinach
Black-eyed Beans	White Beans	Seitan	Oatmeal	Tempeh	Chickpeas
Peanut Butter	Lentils	Amaranth	Almonds	Kidney Beans	Flax Seeds

Ultraviolet light is the invisible radiation in sunlight. "Sunlight may trigger a Lupus rash and it can also trigger symptoms of joint pain and fatigue. Lupus is a disease that goes through periods of quiet and periods of increased disease activity called flares. Many people with lupus experience flares if they get too much sun exposure.

Because most people with lupus are photosensitive and sunlight can trigger symptoms from skin rashes to internal organ damage, protecting yourself from sun exposure is a vital part of lupus management. It's important to know how ultraviolet light from the sun and other sources may stimulate an autoimmune response. Make sure you use a sunscreen of at least 15 SPF and that you are using enough sunscreen to get complete protection.

Here are more tips for protecting sun-sensitive skin:
*Avoid any prolonged sun exposure but be especially careful at mid-day, when ultraviolet light is strongest. Remember that clouds do not filter out all the ultraviolet rays of the sun.
*Most people apply less sunscreen than they need. To achieve the maximum SPF, you need to apply at least one ounce of sunscreen per application. The most frequently missed areas are the back, the sides of the neck, and around the ears.
*Sunlight is not the only source of ultraviolet light. Fluorescent lights and photocopiers emit some ultraviolet light. Tanning beds are not safe for people with lupus.
*Some antibiotics, like tetracycline, can make you more sensitive to sunlight, so ask your doctor or pharmacist about photosensitivity any time you start a new drug.
*Car and house windows screen out UVB rays but not UVA. You can buy films to coat these windows for UVA protection.

UV PROTECTION CHART

Low (0-2)	Medium (3-5)	High (6-7)	Very High (7-10)	Extremely High (11+)
Sunscreen	Sunscreen	Sunscreen	Sunscreen	Sunscreen
Sunglasses	Sunglasses	Sunglasses	Sunglasses	Sunglasses
	Hat	Hat	Hat	Hat
		Shade	Shade	Shade
				Staying indoors between 10am-4pm

Battling Hair Loss

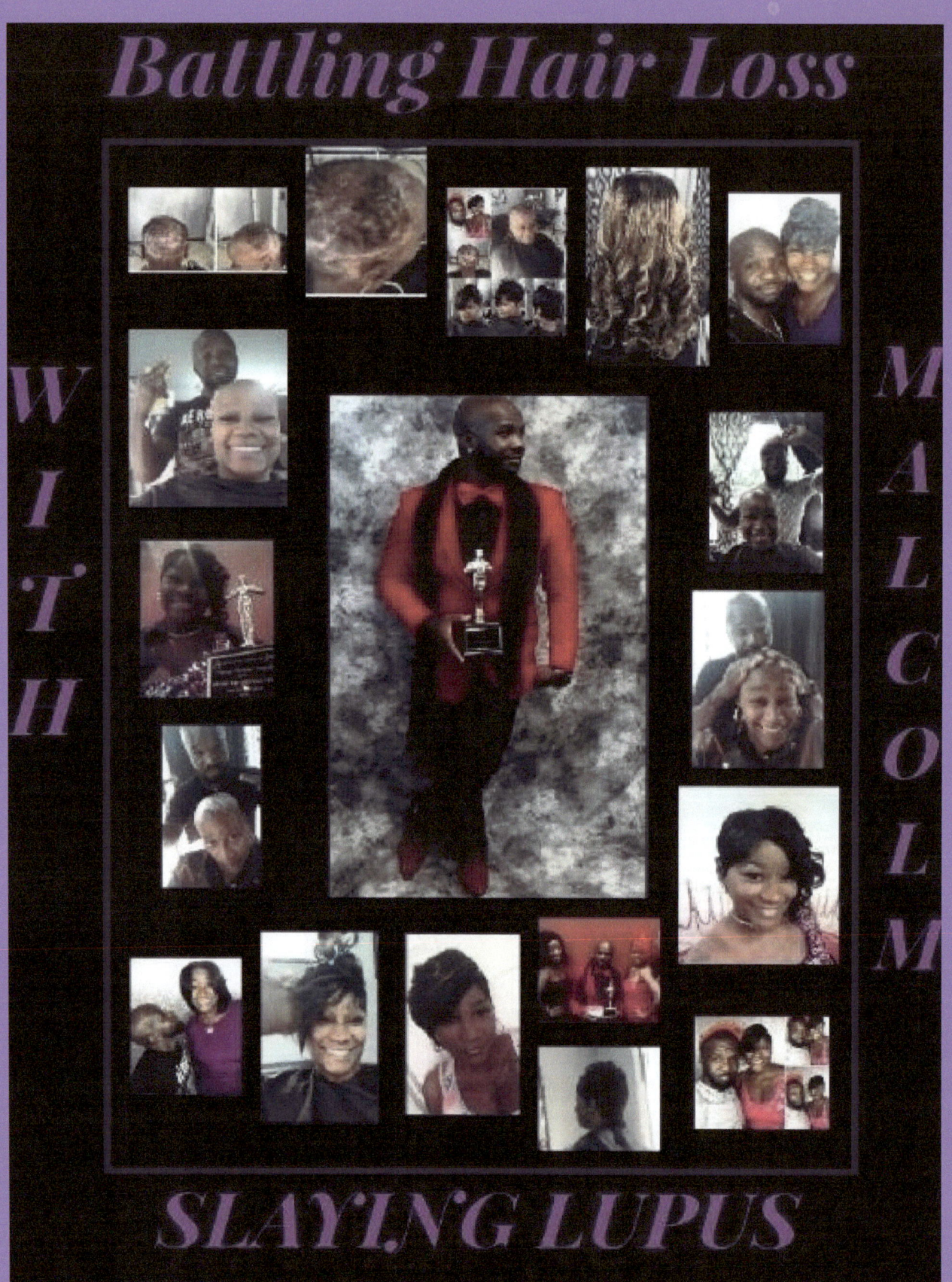

WITH

MALCOLM

SLAYING LUPUS

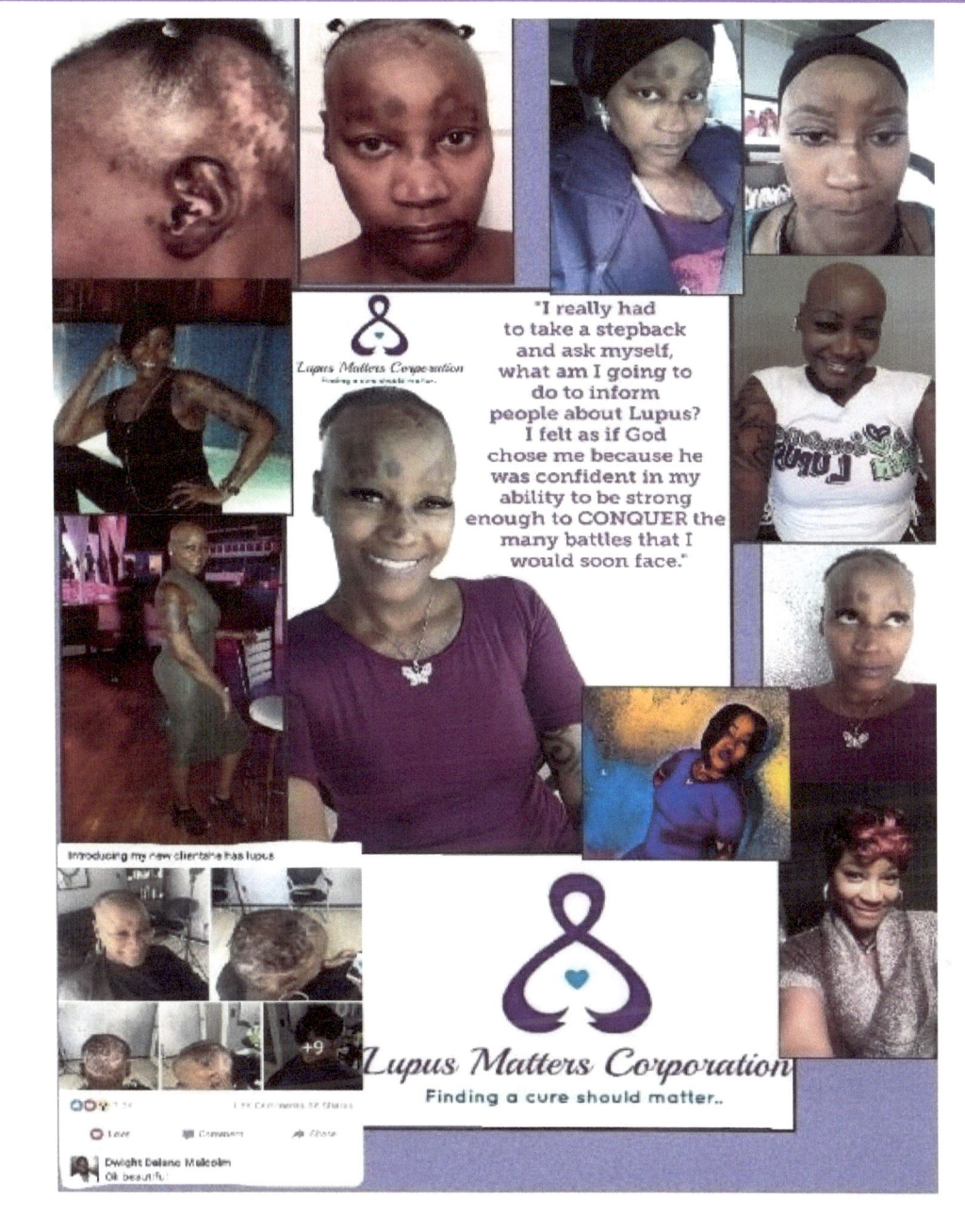

I met Malcolm on September 16th, 2016

I had been following him on social media two weeks prior to me inboxing him.

Story goes like this:

Me: "Hey Dwight if you can do my hair today I promise you I can pay you on the 3rd of October. I just saw your post and I figured it don't hurt to ask can you do something with this jacked up head"

Malcolm: "Come in boo 2107 Faulkner Rd Atlanta Georgia 30324"

Me: "Omgggg thank you thank you thank you can I come at 12"

Malcolm: "Yes"

There goes the start of our relationship.

Getting to know Malcolm, I've learned that although he has gone through a tremendous amount of pain, he continues to remain humble and gives all of his accomplishments to the Lord. I love the fact that he is a God fearing young man. Some of Malcolm's client's hair issues range from hair loss due to Lupus, Diabetes, Cancer and sometimes even stress but he understands that sometimes his clients can't afford to get slayed but Mr. Malcolm has blessed so many people by simply just working with the budget that they have. That can make a person's confidence skyrocket. Someone may enter feeling anxious but by the time Malcolm finishes SLAYING them, they exude sexiness, poise and a boldness that should be rewarded.
In November, Malcolm celebrated a BIG win. He won the Odyssey "Destiny" Award for Best Male Hair Designer 2016. It was well deserved. Way to go Sir, you are an AWESOME soul. Contact Malcolm for all your hair needs.

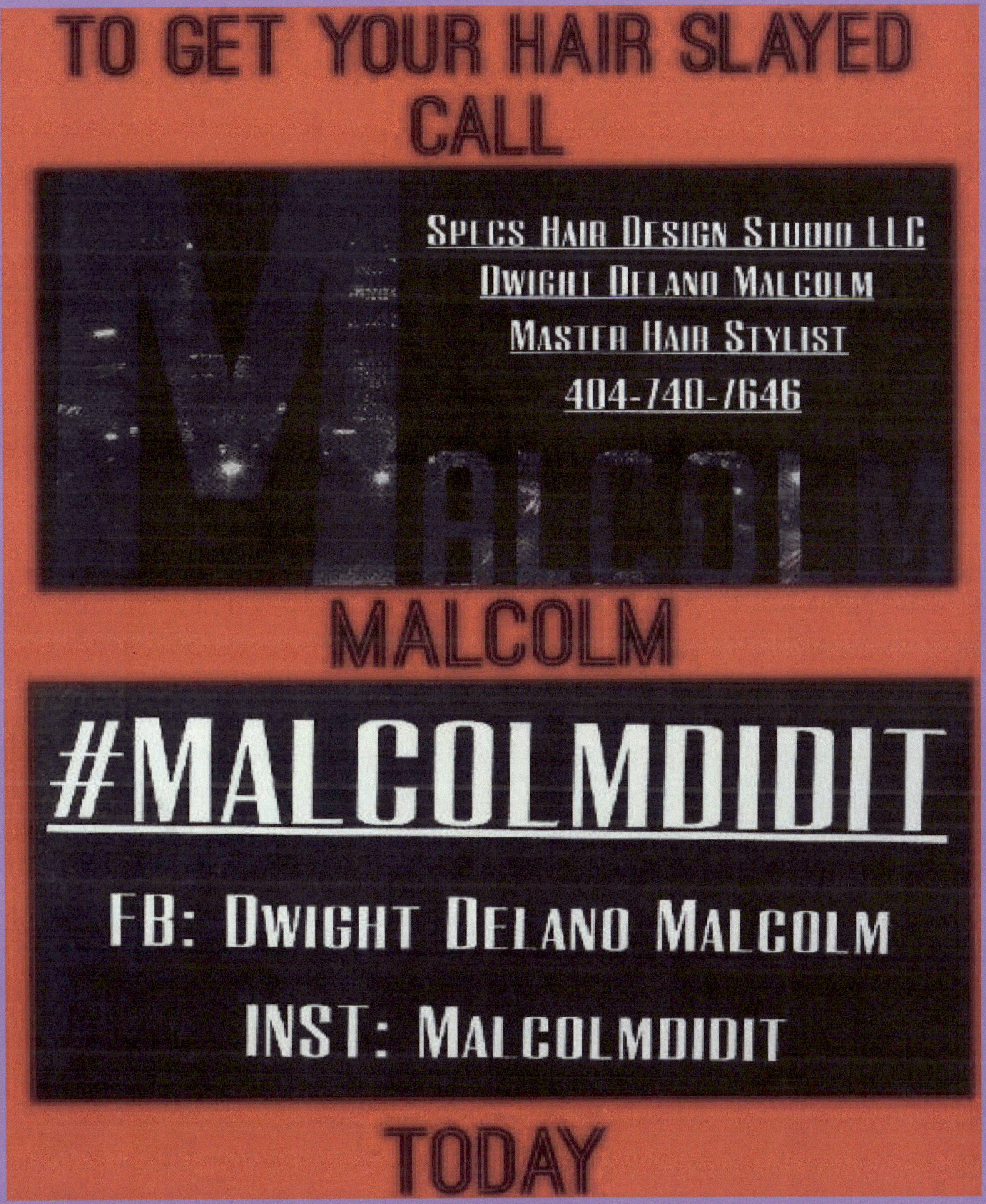
TO GET YOUR HAIR SLAYED
CALL
SPECS HAIR DESIGN STUDIO LLC
DWIGHT DELANO MALCOLM
MASTER HAIR STYLIST
404-740-7646
MALCOLM
MALCOLM
#MALCOLMDIDIT
FB: DWIGHT DELANO MALCOLM
INST: MALCOLMDIDIT
TODAY

Lupus Matters Word Search

```
Y E W N N I S E L N N G P D S
L U O O N U M U P O M U T I I
F G L B P O F M I L R L D S M
R I F U R N I S U P G L K C J
E T L X I I S S L N O W V O K
T A U A F I G E S H E Z D I B
T F P F M S Y S T E M I C D L
U K S E K I D N E Y R A S H M
B E R W N O I T A R O P R O C
T R S D E L S J C L S M E K R
N R L A L L V C G O E Y B D I
I E A N E U L S R E T T A M B
O Z E E K S N I R S X K V E B
J S W S H Q I G N N I A R B O
S S T Y M Y B D Z G R Q H S N
```

BUTTERFLY
DISCOID
FATIGUE
IMMUNE
LUNG
PAINFUL
REMISSION
SWELLING

BRAIN
DEPRESSION
DLE
ILLNESS
KIDNEY
MATTERS
RASH
SLE
WOLF

CORPORATION
DISEASE
HEART
JOINT
LUPUS
PURPLE
RIBBON
SYSTEMIC

LMC NEWS

Looking for actors
no experience needed
Auditions Coming Soon

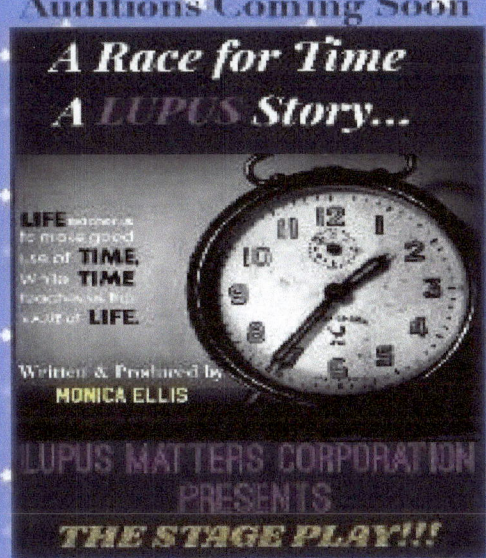

Submit your
story today?

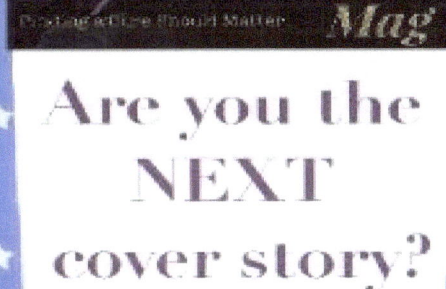

Are you the
NEXT
cover story?

Follow us
on Facebook

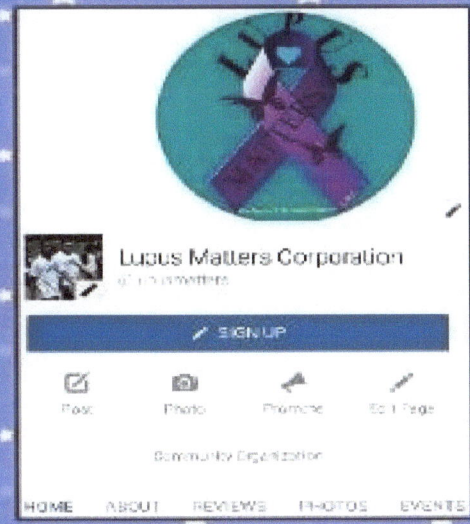

Email for details & pricing

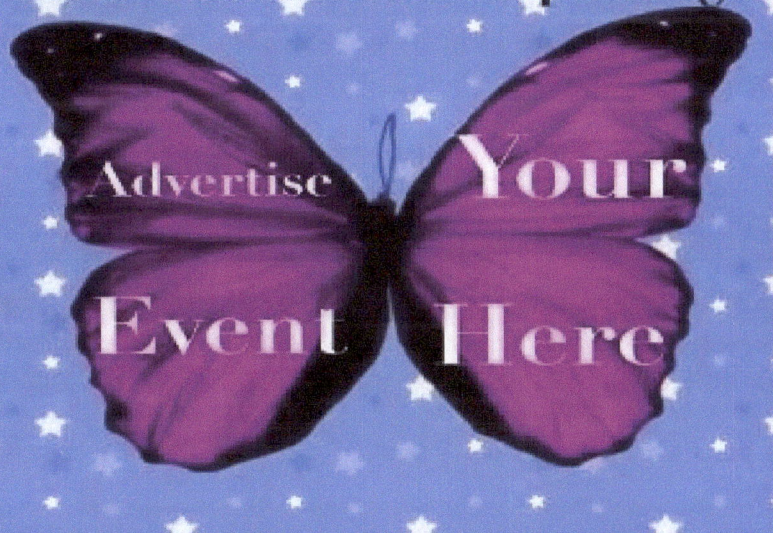

Advertise Your
Event Here

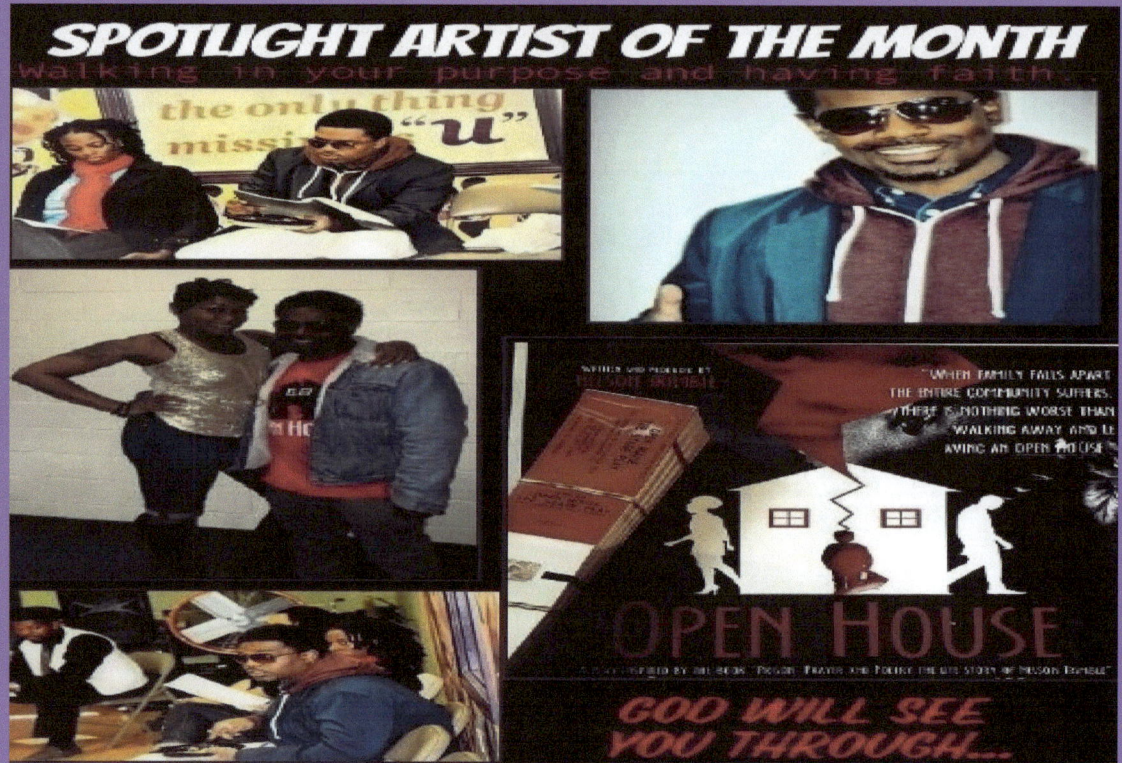

Nelson "SPARATIC" Trimble ~ The General Sparatic

His words are raw, real and relevant. I met Sparatic in 2015 and I found myself being motivated and encouraged by his movement **Families Unified Strength in One Number** {FUSION} of promoting Reading, the Arts and Entrepreneurship. FUSION's moto is Saving Kids Lives One Book at a Time.

I find that Mr. SPARATIC, is very passionate about his work, his faith and preserving his energy for positivity. I chose this young man not because I know him but because he is a great example of how to stand tall and proud after the obstacles in life knock you down. He's been through so much and still has risen above it all, to become a Producer, Director, Author, Motivational Speaker, a Playwright and first and foremost a Spoken Word Artist. He's an advocator for Autism, Diabetes & Lupus. "*You must be the change you want to see in the world*". *Mahatma Gandhi &* my friend you certainly are.

Be Sure to follow "Fusion Movement", "Open House" and Nelson Trimble on Facebook
To get date for the OPEN HOUSE Stageplay and other events.

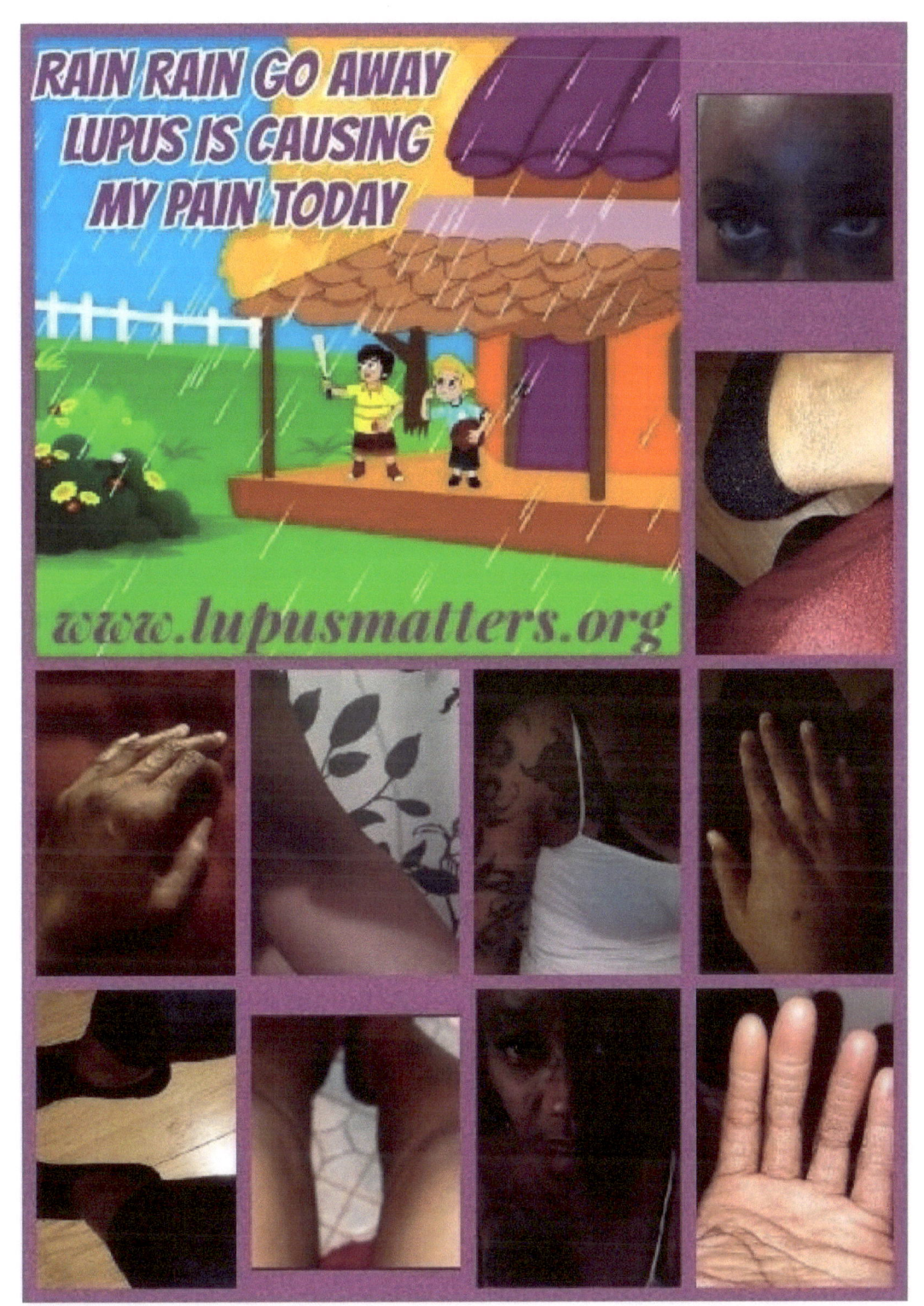

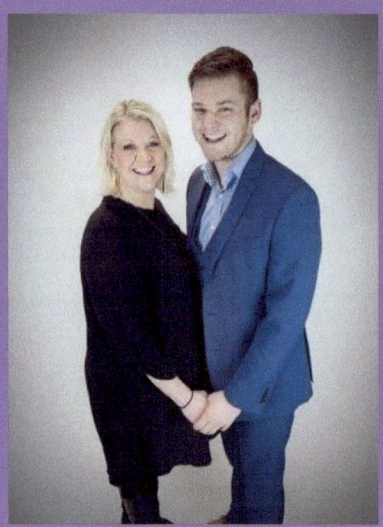

Dondra L. Kinna

iResearch Atlanta

T: 404.537.1281

M: 770.378.3927

www.iResearchAtlanta.com

Zach Mitchell-Recruitment Specialist

Starting as a Market Researcher in 2014 at UWG paved the foundation for his transition to working at iResearch Atlanta, as part of the recruitment team. As a Recruitment Specialist, he participates in recruiting patients, administering intakes, managing all data collection pertaining to subjects and screening outcomes, maintaining information related to all active studies, coordinate consent process, educating and providing information to patients and families pertaining to clinical trials.

--

Dondra Kinna-Recruitment Specialist

Began her career as an Intake Coordinator at a research site in the Atlanta area. She Participated in Intake administration, managed appointments, coordinated activities and outings for patients, responded to all calls/ messages for site specific research, educated potential subjects on all active studies. Formed and maintained relationships with the local community and Health affiliates.

Together, Dondra and Zach have built strong long lasting relationships with many different local affiliates and nonprofit organizations. These connections stretch from Human Sex Trafficking support groups to Senior living facilities. They have a tremendous amount of support from local community shelters, advocacy groups and ministries from their efforts to stay involved within the community. Dondra and Zach are always "on", ready to tell others about iResearch Atlanta and how important research is for everyone in the community. They are consistently educating groups, families, and volunteers about research. And how it can be beneficial in hopes of breaking the stigma of mental health and research.

What is Clinical Research?

Through the remarkable work of doctors and scientists, new drugs are being created every year to treat a wide range of disorders and diseases. After many experiments, the final stage of the testing process is to have real people with the specific condition try the medication. Since everyone's body is a little different, this is a critical step to understanding how the new medication will affect the general population, and most importantly, how effective it really is.

Sometimes this step proves that a promising new drug isn't as good as it seems. Other times, it proves that the new medication has miraculous effects.

As with any research, there are risks. For many participants, the hope of having significant relief makes those risks worthwhile. We'll be more than happy to outline the specific risks associated with the program you are interested in so that you can make the right decision for you.

It's natural to have questions. Get the answers you need to feel comfortable.

What are the risks and benefits of a research program?

Will it cost me anything? Do I get compensated?

How long does it take?

Will I be treated by real doctors?

What happens when I sign up?

Have more questions? Get in touch.

Ready to join? Check out our Current Programs.

What if I have a medical problem while in the program?

Get the answers to these questions and more details about our new *LUPUS* trial by logging onto:

www.iresearchatlanta.com

H.P. **Acthar** GEL
(repository corticotropin injection) 80 U/mL

For
SYSTEMIC LUPUS
ERYTHEMATOSUS (LUPUS)

Acthar is a prescription medicine for flares or on a regular basis (maintenance) in people with systemic lupus erythematosus (lupus).

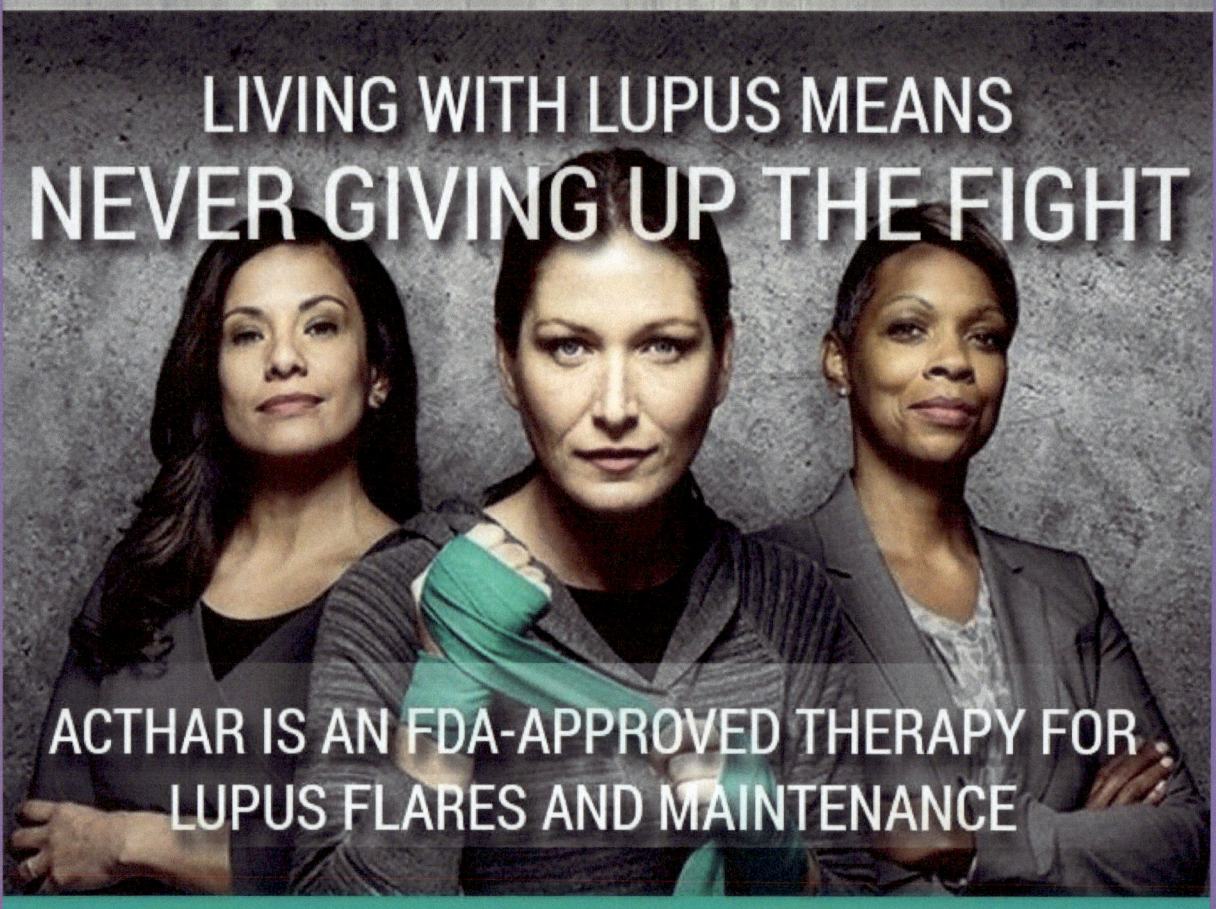

LIVING WITH LUPUS MEANS
NEVER GIVING UP THE FIGHT

ACTHAR IS AN FDA-APPROVED THERAPY FOR LUPUS FLARES AND MAINTENANCE

Is Acthar right for me?

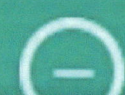

Important Safety Information

Who should NOT *take Acthar?*

You should **not take** Acthar if you have:

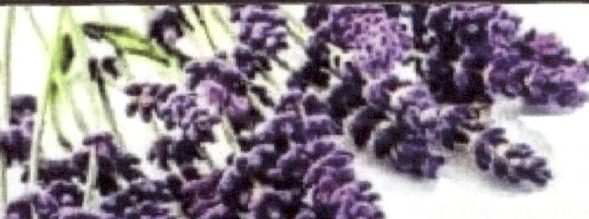
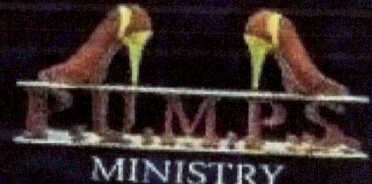

MONICA ELLIS'
STRUGGLE'S
WITH
DISCOID LUPUS

LUPUS ADVOCATE, AUTHOR & ENTREPRENEUR, SHUNS AWAY THE STIGMA OF HAVING DISCOID LUPUS. WHILE LIVING LIFE TO THE FULLEST...

BY JACKIE FOOTE

THERE IS ONE WORD TO DESCRIBE MONICA ELLIS, 42.

INSPIRING !!!

I've interviewed quite a few people in preparation of my interview with Ms. Ellis and I must say that the word inspiration came up fairly often. She has been hailed a SHE-RO to some and a warrior to most but to her, she is just an average girl trying to survive what most people would crumble from.

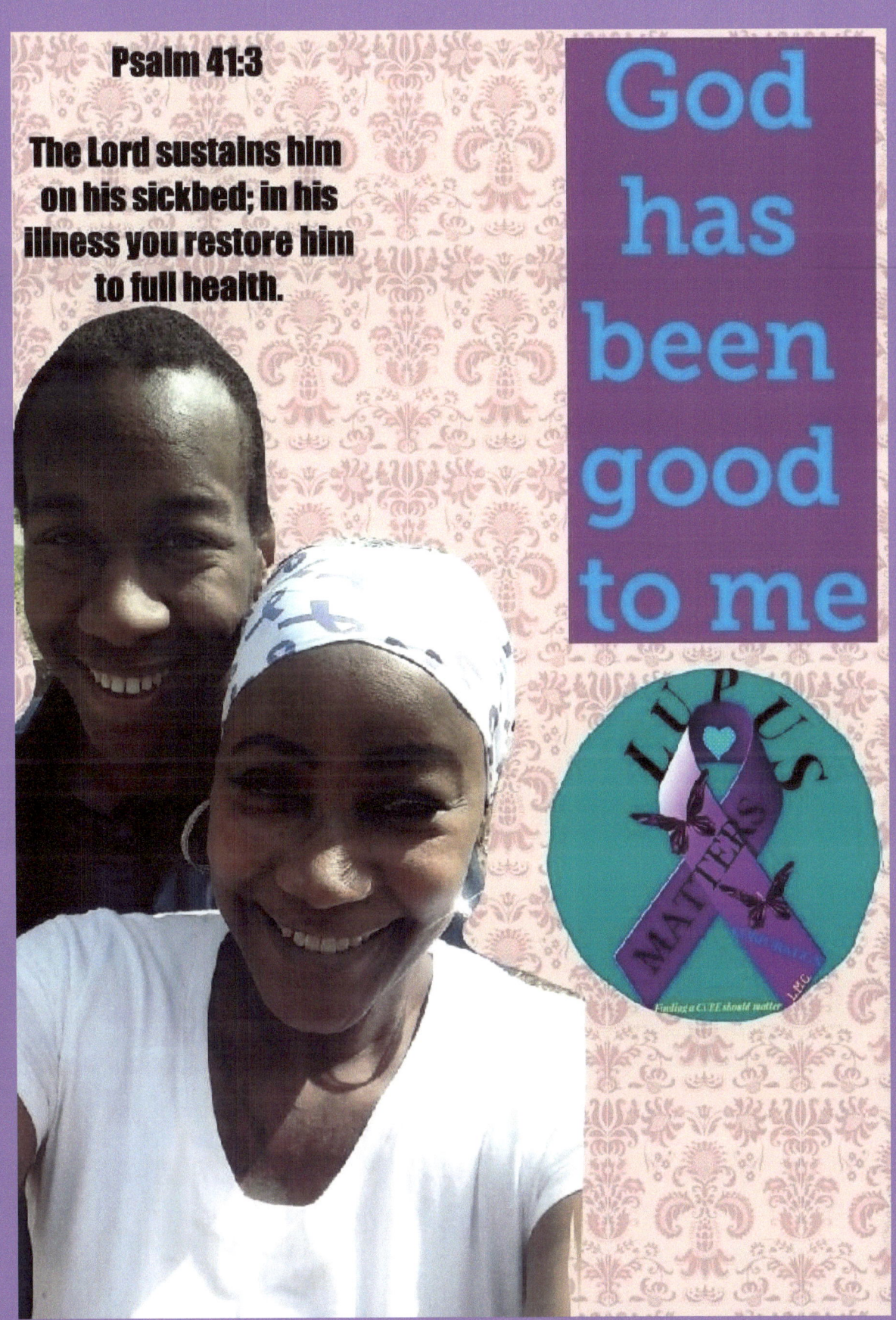

Psalm 41:3

The Lord sustains him on his sickbed; in his illness you restore him to full health.

God has been good to me

LUPUS MATTERS

Finding a CURE should matter

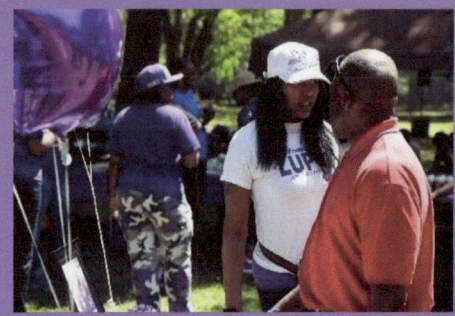

Monica, advocating and Educating others about Lupus...

Monica, was born in Detroit, Michigan & raised in Miami, Fl. She founded Lupus Matters Corporation in 2007 after being diagnosed with discoid lupus and shortly thereafter systemic lupus in 2001. Monica has 16 years in the lupus community. She has served all these years battling and surviving this illness. During this time, she was laying the foundation to create Lupus Matters Corporation.

Although being a mother of one son was very challenging, she could not give up her fight to live and raise her son.

Kidney issues, peripheral neuropathy, pleurisy and other symptoms that caused her near-death experiences, motivated her to live life to the fullest. Monica has been awarded:

*The 2015 Jackie Tally Lupus fighter award by Blaq Pearl entertainment

*The bronze level award for raising over $599 by Alliance for Lupus Association

*The bronze-level over $1,500 by Alliance for Lupus Association
*Just recently, Lupus Matters Corporation has been presented with the proclamation for May 2016 to Proclaim that may be Lupus Awareness Month for the Cities of Conyers and Cartersville Georgia.

*Monica is a published author of the book Some People Kill Me, Living My Life with Lupus.
*The 2015 Savory vegan calendar, after becoming vegan in 2011.

* She is a song writer and lyricist of the hit single "Ta All My Lupie Chix" the Lupus Matters anthem.

* Lupus Matters Corporation is set to release the first edition of their magazine Lupus Matters Magazine in May of 2017

*She is a member of the Cliff Hangaz BC

*She has also founded the Lupie Riderz MC

Monica started to get little ringworm-like lesions all over her skin. These lesions started to scare her scalp, chest, legs, ears and face as well as other parts of her body. She felt ugly, alone and trapped. To make matters worse, when her hair started to fall out, she was scared as to what people may say about her. She felt that she would look like and old lady if she wore wigs. She was in her prime and too young to feel this old. She went into depression for a while until one day on a carnival cruise in 2009 she decided after months of contemplating to shave her head bald, slap on some big bold hoop earrings and a cute sundress and that was the beginning of her confidence to LIVE LIFE TO THE FULLEST!!! She began to understand the beauty in herself and if she didn't feel it, no one could feel it for her. She realized the she was not her hair or lack thereof, her ugly skin marks or the depression that kept her captive for such a long time. She became more vocal about Discoid Lupus and the affects that it can have on a person emotional state of mind (IF they let it). Monica, tells me that the advice the she would tell anyone going through such a devastating diagnosis, is to talk to God, keep him first in all things. She also says that it's not the end of the world, never let what people think about you dictate your success in life. She say's life is what you make it, so

"*If living life to the fullest is the mission, we* **should** *be in remission*".

Monica, is just thankful for that love that God has giving her to continue to live, advocate & educated others about this terrible disease.

Because, finding a cure should matter...

Lupus Matters Corporation

Finding a cure should matter..

KickRocksLupus

After becoming friends with this beautiful butterfly, a year ago, we finally had the pleasure of meeting at a mutual friend's book signing. It was like we knew each other for years. She was as lovely in person as she was in her social media pictures. I personally feel that as we grow older, meeting people takes on a new meaning, you will either have a friend for life or have someone that was only meant to be there for a short time. I look forward to a great friendship with her.

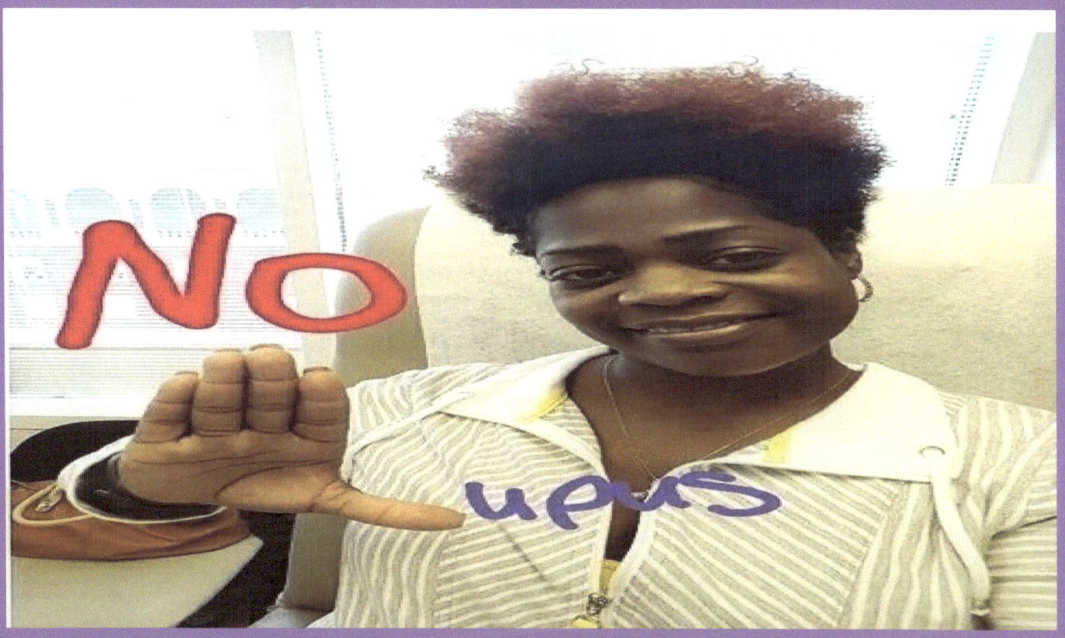

I was a healthy 40-years-old mother of three awesome kids. Living life day to day like everyone else. Going to work, taking care of the kids, and enjoying life. So, I thought. Then it hit me like a Mack truck, BOOM! My life as I knew it changed. I was diagnosed with lupus nephritis and stage 5 kidney failure. I hadn't been feeling well for some time and just assumed I had the worst case of the flu ever. I was vomiting, cold sweats, fevers, loss of appetite, dark urine, decrease in urine and extreme fatigue. One night after being off work for more than two weeks I thought I was going to go in and decided to take my oldest daughter who is 18 with me. Impossible because I worked for federal agency so employees only. I wasn't in my right state of mind. We ended up a hospital more than forty minutes away. During my wait in the ER I may have gotten up to go to the bathroom nearly ten times with no urine passing. Soon it was my turn to be seen. I was asked to give a urine sample. I couldn't pee, I was told that I would have to have a catheter put in me, in order to get a urine, drop. After being unsuccessful in getting any urine this is when all hell broke loose. After all the questions, taking blood, poking and prodding I was admitted as a patient. I was told within hours that I was at stage 5 kidney failure. Are you talking to me? What did this mean? Then I was told I had Lupus Nephritis. Ok what happens next? I was given aggressive steroids to try and stop the lupus from attacking my kidneys any further. I had to go on dialysis that next morning because I wasn't passing urine on my own. Toxin was building up in my body. While in the hospital I was scared, and confused and needed to talk to my aunt who had been battling lupus for over fifteen years. She gave me some advice and encouraged me to research the illness on my own. This disease became a life changing moment that I had not prepared for. I was not prepared for the financial stress. I was out of work for nearly four months and had exhausted all my sick and donated leave, as well as friends and family. Fortunately, by the grace of God my kidneys reverted and I could stop dialysis and return to work. For the next two and a half months I played catch up with bill collectors but could never catch up. I had only been back at work two months when I woke up one morning and my eyes had swollen. They were so swollen and red it look as if though I had a bad allergic reaction to something. I ended up going to the ER because it was the weekend and my doctor's office was closed.

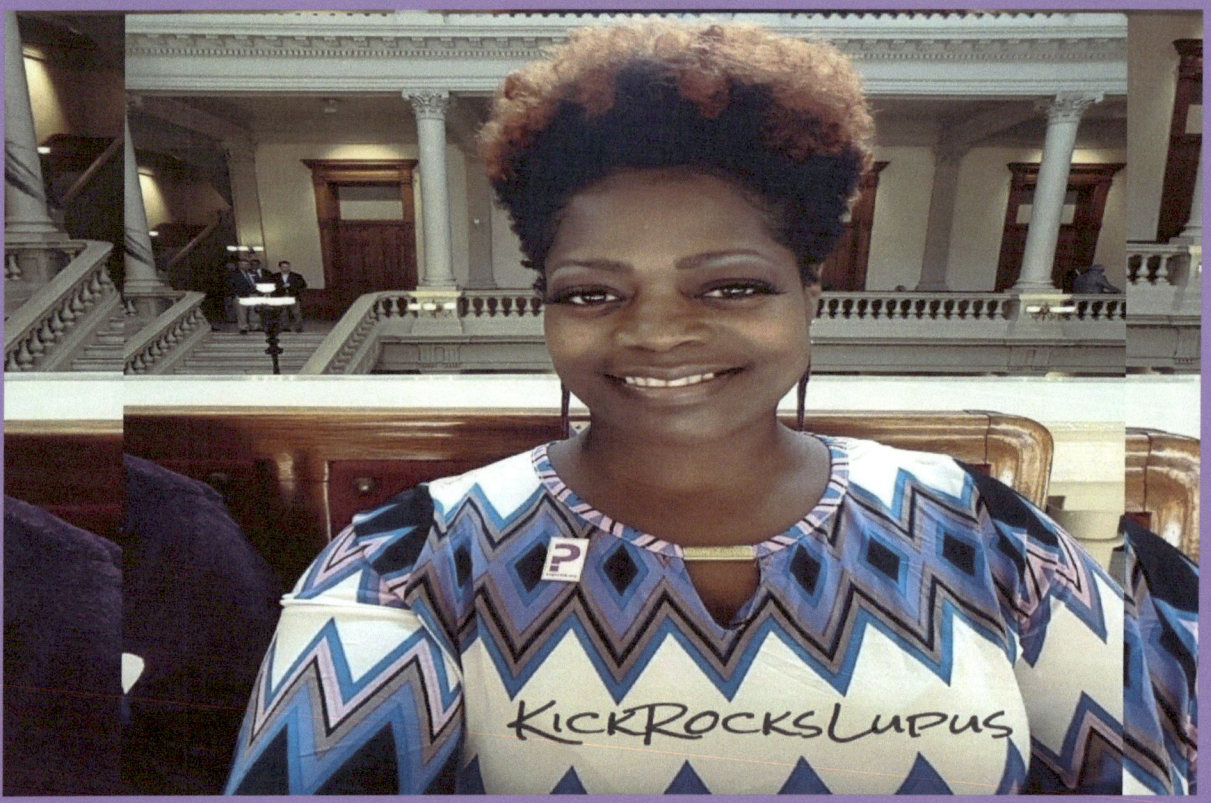

I was told I had contracted Conjunctivitis. I was also told after some urine and blood work had come back that my creatinine level was off, protein was in my urine and my hemoglobin was a little low but not low enough for a blood transfusion. The doctor contacted my nephrologist and they decided that I didn't need to be admitted now. I had a follow up appointment with my nephrologist a few days later to discuss the results of my 24-hour urinalysis test I had done the week before. During my visit, I was placed back on steroids and one of my other meds, cellcept, were increased in dosage. That same day after leaving my doctors I stopped by a good friends' place of business to visit. After only twenty minutes of being there I began to develop a sharp pain in my abdomen that caused me to take a trip to the ER via EMS. Once again after all the drawing of blood, urine samples and more poking and prodding lupus was attacking my kidneys. I had to be transported to a sister hospital where specialist was on staff. My stay this time was a little over a week. It has been very hard since I haven't been able to work so no income and once the filing process of anything started it's a waiting game. I recently filed early retirement disability and SSI... I know good luck with that. I was a mechanic so with all my ailments that occur due to lupus I was unable to perform my work duties.

After being out of work for nearly a year, the struggle was real, I was given early retirement. My husband and my kids had been my strength through my battles with this disease.   Once I put my 'Big Girl Panties' on and changed my mindset thing started to change for the better in my life. In March of 2013 I went into business for myself by opening a cleaning company. I like to clean, but I love the result of having a clean house.   It's something I can control whether I choose to accept a job or not. Months later I invested in a career to become a Credit Restoration Agent.   My husband and I needed to restore our credit. After learning so much about my rights I decided to become an agent. It only made sense because I knew of others that were in the same situation that we were.   Having three streams of income now felt good. It just motivated me more to want to have more. Now I am in the process of going back to taking my real estate class to become a realtor as I set out to do back in 2007. Life may have changed for me in a way I would have never thought, but I could not allow lupus to take over my life. I had to do something besides being consumed with pity and depression. God and the universe has had a plan for me before my creation, and I believe it is to inspire others.

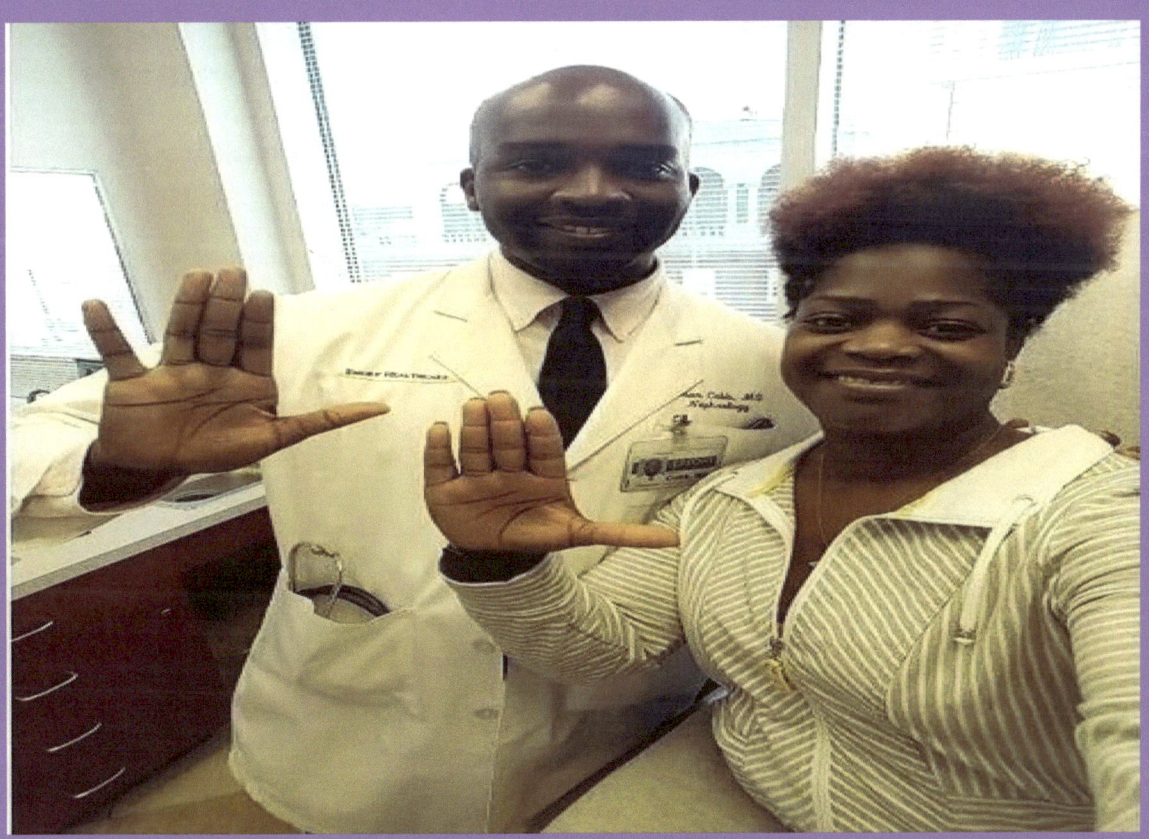

NO LIMITS TO LUPUS LIVING

Count your health by thrills not pills

People with late onset lupus have a good survival rate and rarely die of the disease or complications of therapy when treated conservatively.

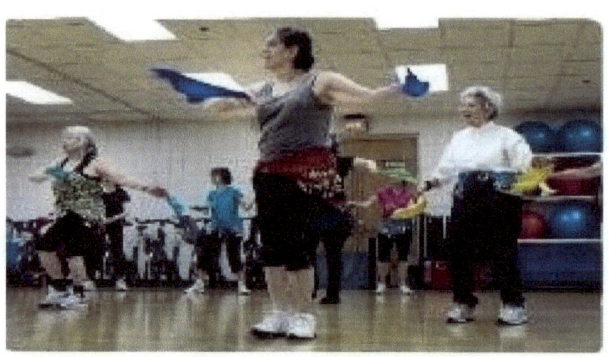

"Diagnosis in the Elderly. It is very difficult to diagnose **lupus** in **seniors**. It often gets misdiagnosed or undiagnosed for up to 3 years. ... It is often diagnosed as a rheumatic disease or a drug-induced systemic **lupus** erythematosus (**SLE**)."

The longer you live the more beautiful life becomes!

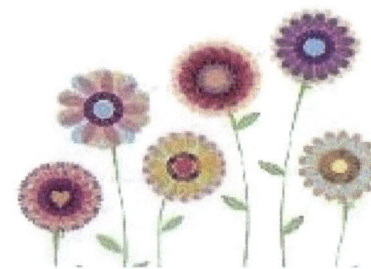

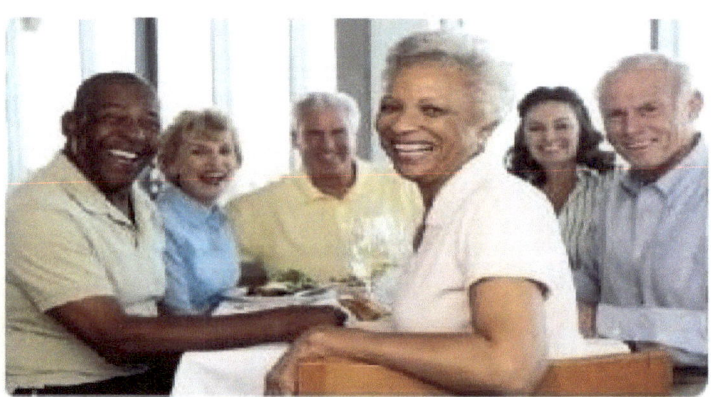

SENIOR CITIZENS WITH LUPUS

About 10-20% of all cases first occur in people ages 50-65. Symptoms like arthritis, fever, serositis, neuropsychiatric symptoms, lung disease and Raynaud's syndrome occur more frequently in elderly patients compared to younger patients, while malar rash, discoid lupus and glomerulonephritis are less common in the elderly than the young.

It is very difficult to diagnose lupus in seniors. It often gets misdiagnosed or undiagnosed for up to 3 years. The good thing about the disease in older people is that the inflammation is less severe which may account for the issues with diagnosing the disease.

Elderly men and women live a more sedentary lifestyle, plus medications taken for lupus like Prednisone can lead to osteoporosis.

The disease is a challenge to manage. Therefore regular checkups to monitor the disease are important.

Eat a healthy
Get annual vaccinations for the flu and pneumonia
Keep blood pressure and cholesterol under control with medication and diet
Monitor osteoporosis development.
Get regular dental care
Get regular eye examinations
Avoid smoking at all costs

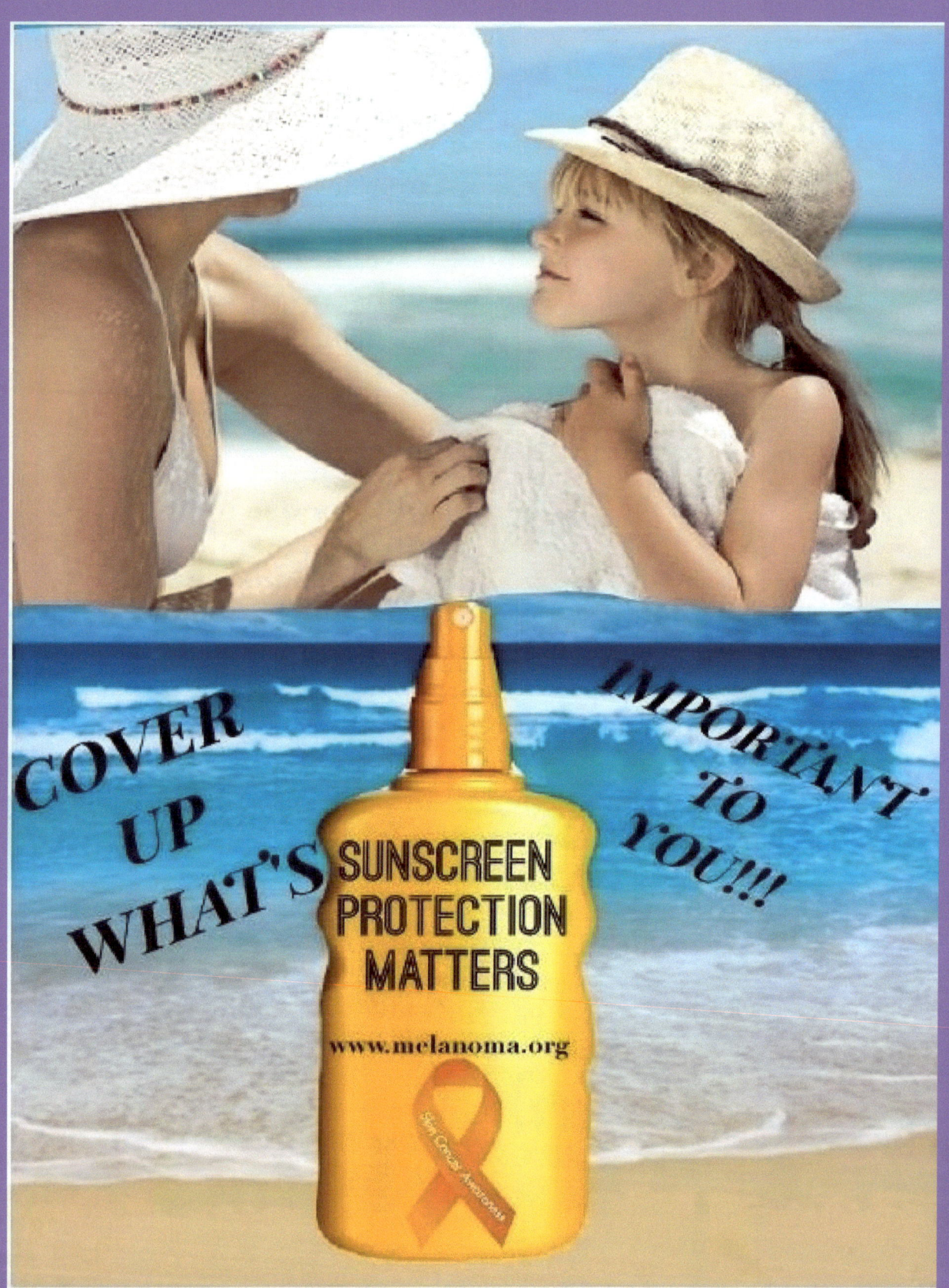

Tanning is a very popular to some and may not be regarded as a serious risk. Some might say it'll never happen to me. But Skin cancer does not pick and choose, it is real and we need to bring awareness to the seriousness of Melanoma Cancer. No matter if it's at the beach, in a tanning bed or from the sun. The UV radiation from either of these are harmful. People who use a tanning bed before the age of 35 increase their risk for Melanoma by 75 percent. As many as 90 percent of Melanomas are estimated to be caused by ultraviolet (UV) exposure. The debate that you can get vitamin D from a tanning bed but truth is all necessary vitamin D can be found in a healthy diet or from vitamin supplement. Consult your doctor if you have any concerns about your vitamin D levels. Melanoma is the most common form of cancer and the leading cause of death in women. There is no such thing as a safe tan, it can lead to age spots, wrinkles, skin cancer and premature aging. There are other methods of tanning, like pills and injections which have additional health risk. One of the best ways to reduce Melanoma is to educate people about the dangers of tanning and early detection and prevention. If we take in consideration that we DON'T have to modify our natural skin to be beautiful. Just embrace the skin that you are in and be confident in it. For more details contact www.melanoma.org

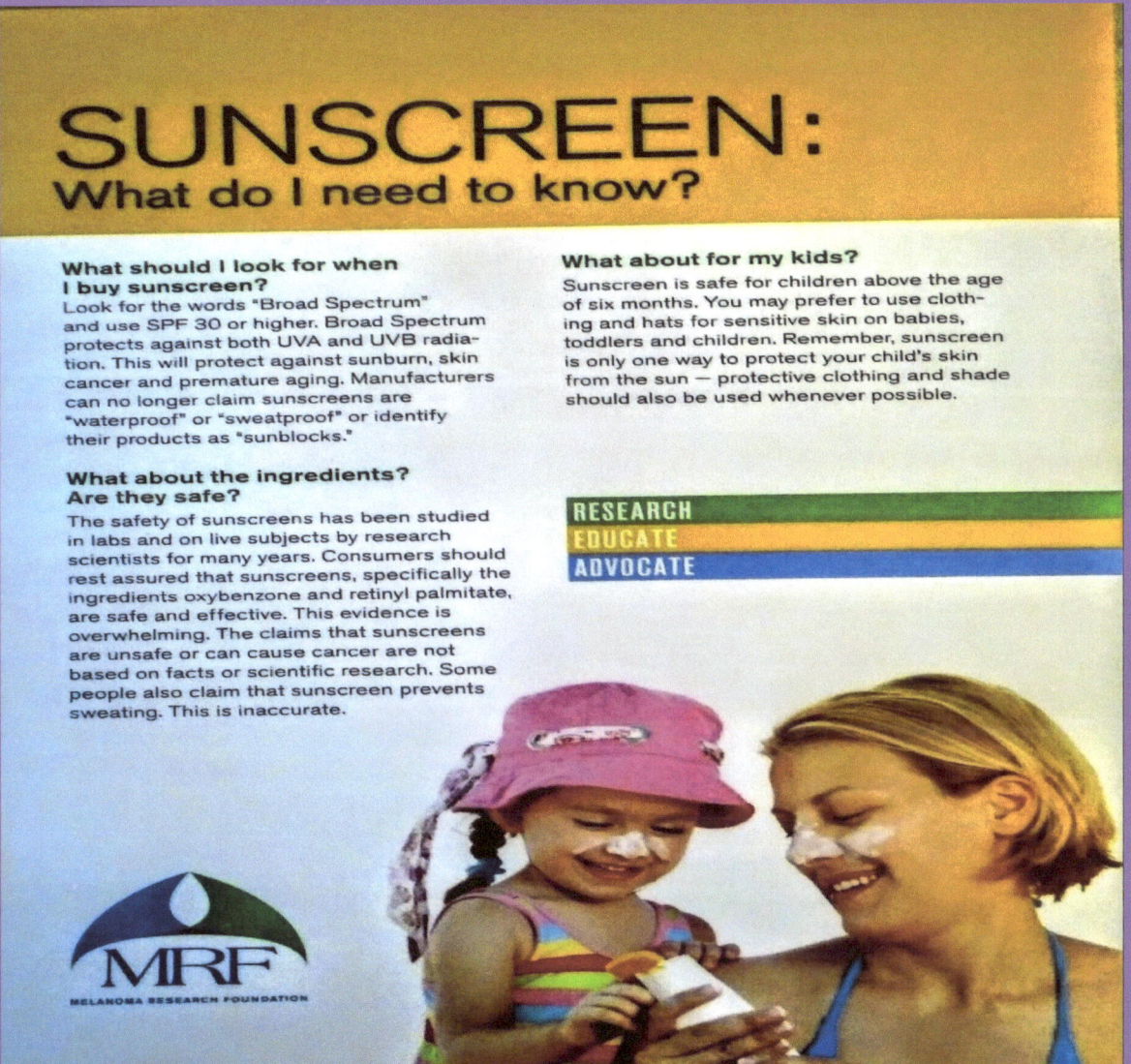

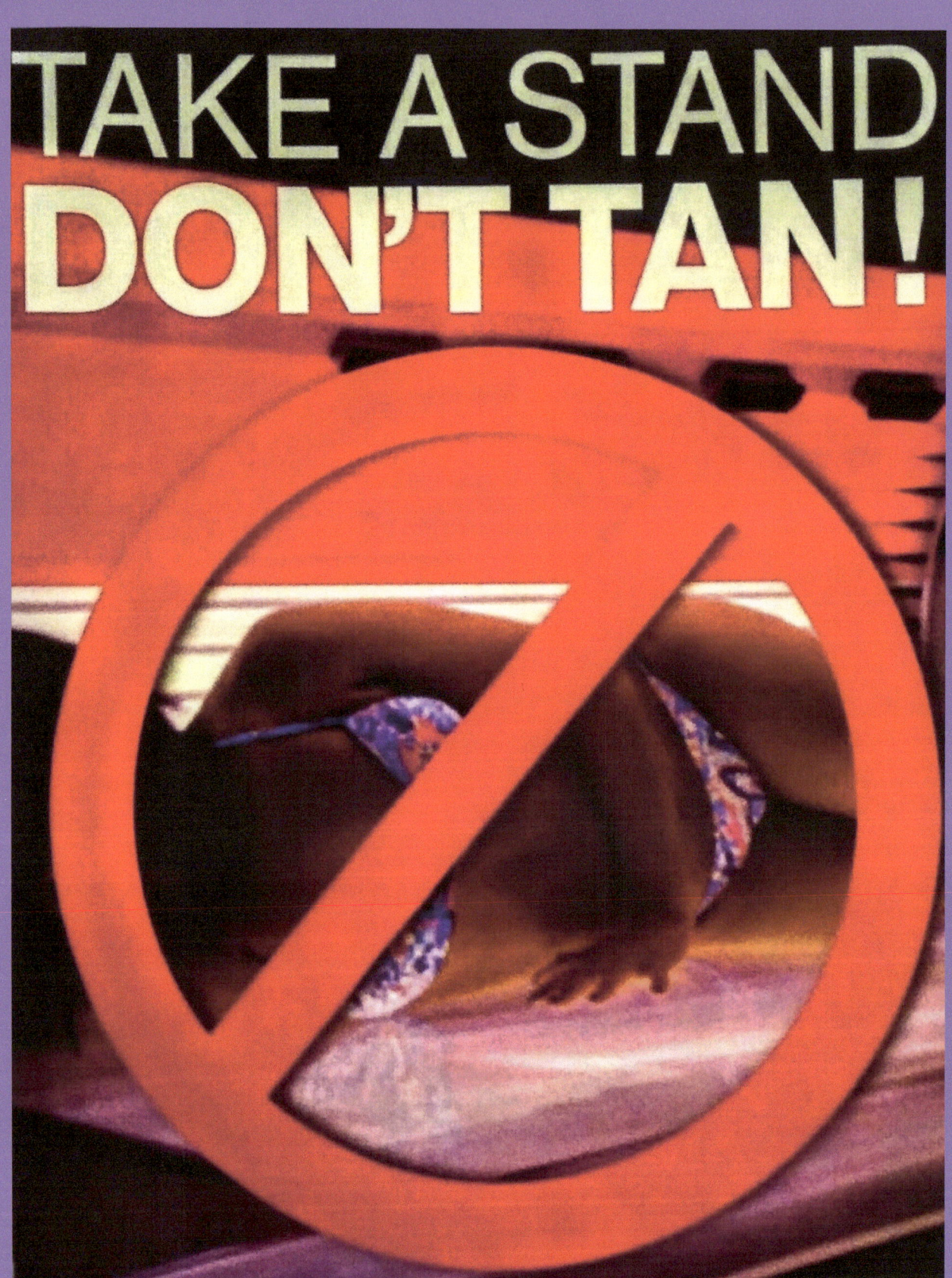

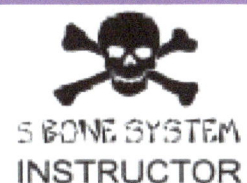
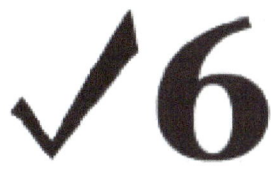
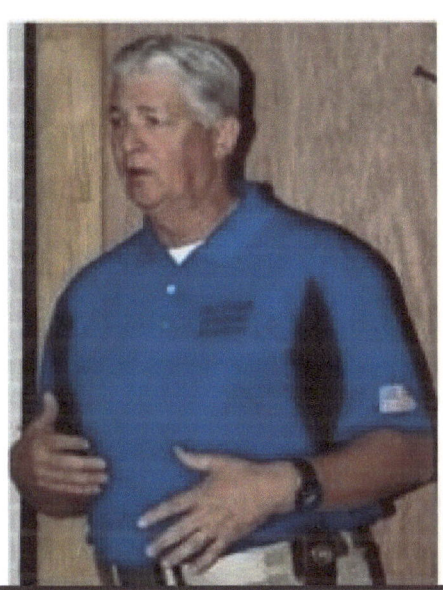
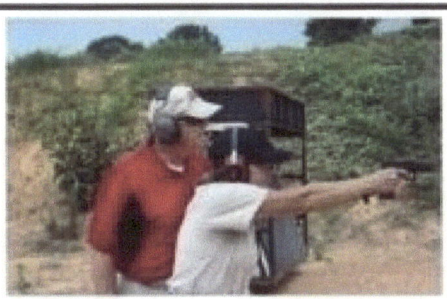

Taco Tuesday
Vegan meal of the day...

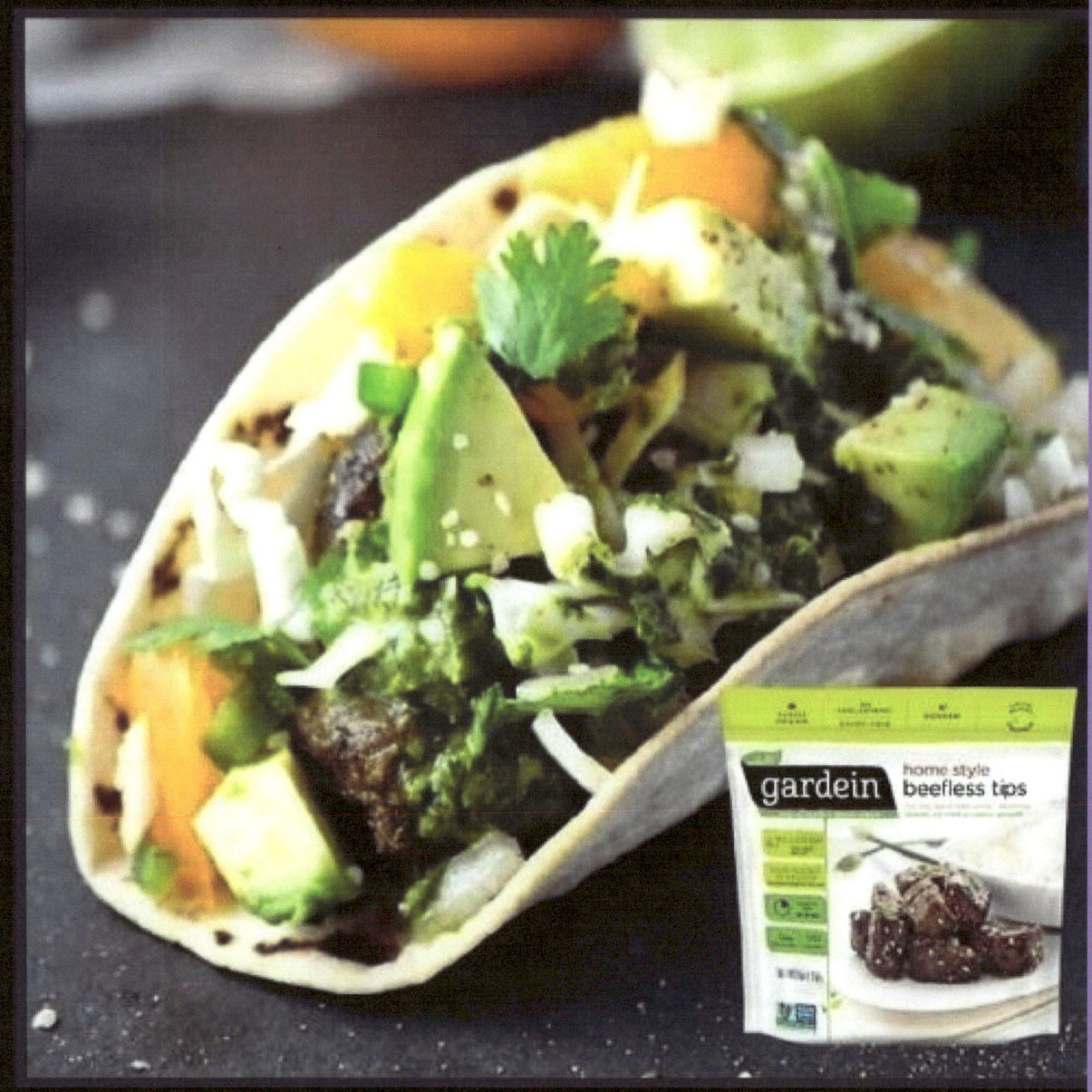

Gardein products are a great meat substitute with plenty of protein...

STARR STATUS

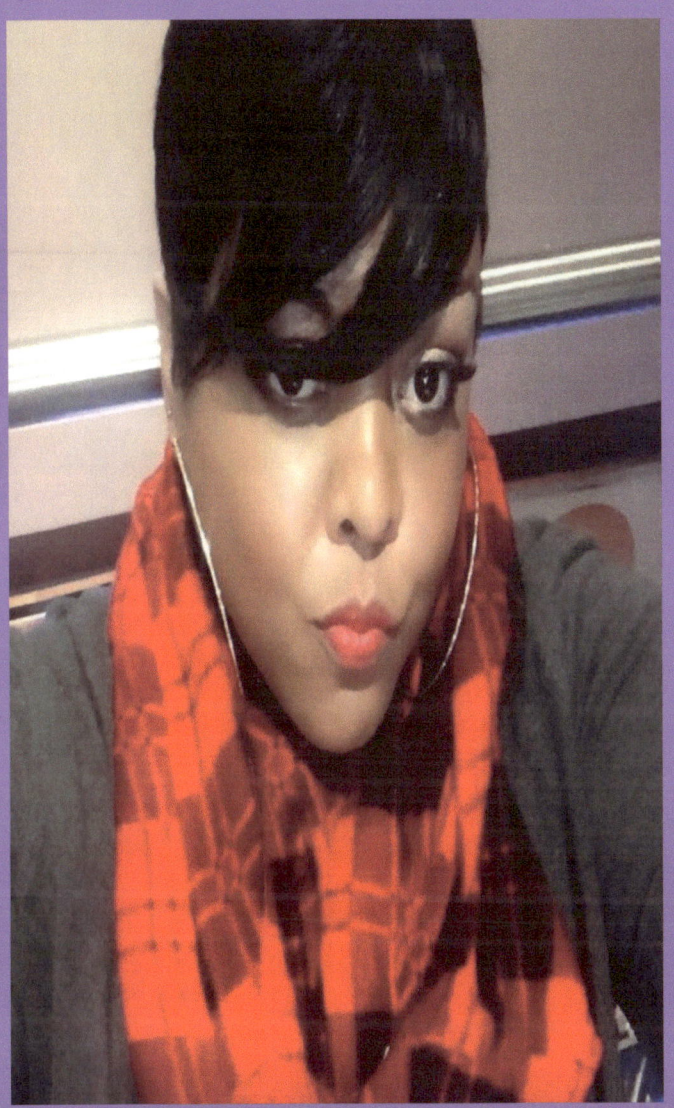 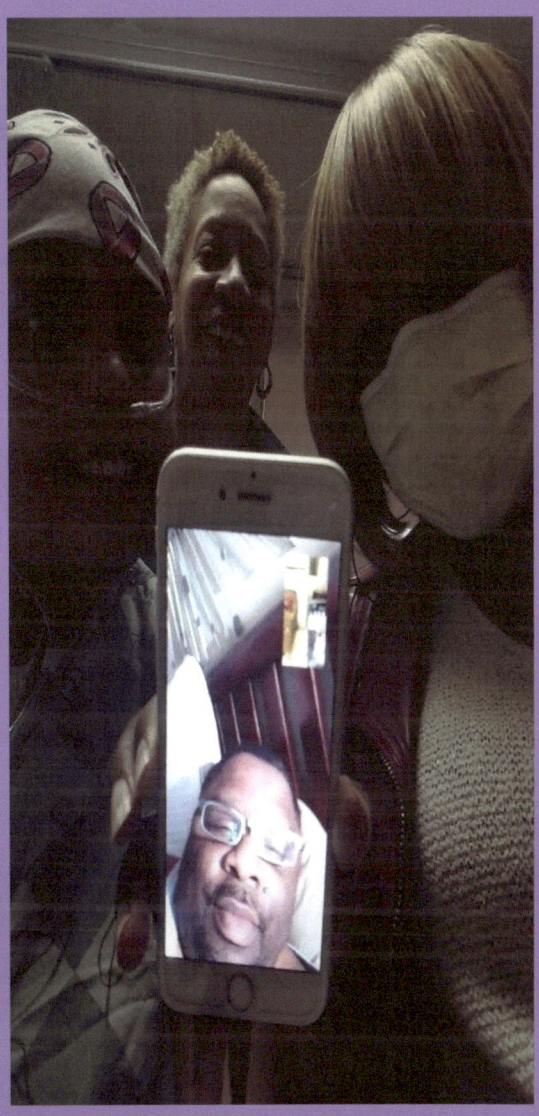

Such a beautiful soul. A woman of God, a wife and a mother. Topaz Henderson, faced Lupus head on and did not give up until the fight was over. Battling Lung disease and Sjögren's Disease, she was a warrior at best. Loving wife, proud mother and trusting friend.

You will truly be missed. R.I.H. *Mrs.Starr*

http://www.glewislupusfoundation.org/

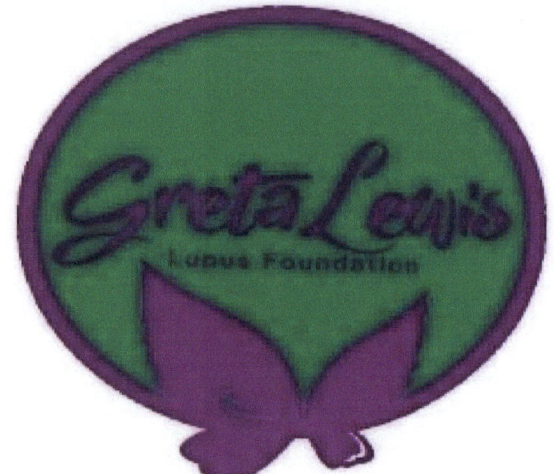

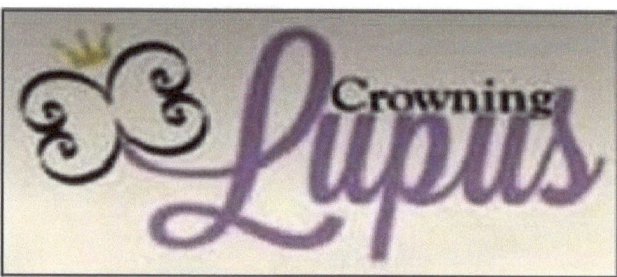

http://www.crowninglupus.com/

Support your
local
Non-Profit
Organizations!!!

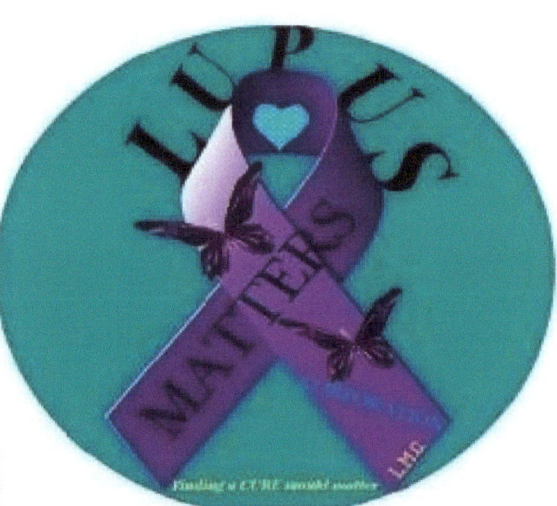

http://lupusmatters.org/

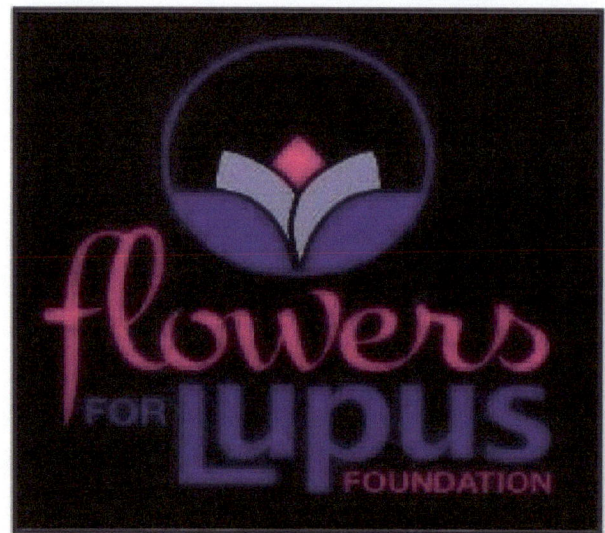

The community
needs them!!

http://www.flowersforlupus.org/

Lovely Lupus

The butterfly of my life has Lupus...

When lupus takes a turn for the worse, all that you hope for is a love that will stand the test of time. A love that will strengthen the bond that you vowed to keep forever. Living with Lupus brings about some difficult challenges and insecurities but the feeling of being in love makes us feel secure, wanted and beautiful. Just as our spouse ensures that we are ok, we want nothing more than to know when our loved one feels overwhelmed or frustrated. We understand that sometimes lupus can be a bit much for our significant others and we never want to feel burdensome to them. But when you're heart is in the right place and your love is unconditional, love will past the test and conquer whatever **LUPUS** throws at us.

World Famous Lupians

Toni Braxton

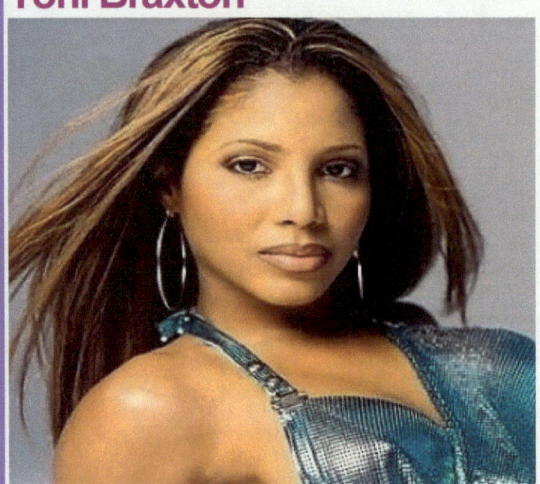

Singer **Toni Braxton** announced she has lupus. While accepting a Women in Achievement award at the 8th Annual Lupus LA Bag Ladies Luncheon, she told the audience: "Today I'm going to talk about it because I'm a survivor and I'm here, and I don't want to lose hope. This is what lupus looks like. "Toni then took to Twitter to share with fans and well-wishers that she feels a "relief" after coming forward.
Thank you, Toni, for realizing that LUPUS MATTERS!!!

Oleta Adams

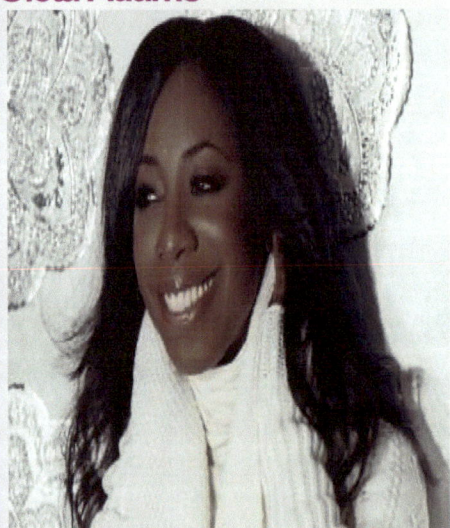

In 2011 Grammy nominated singer **Oleta Adams** told of how she had suffered from lupus for ten years. She said "Lupus has affected every area of my life. We need to bring attention to this disease to further research and development of new treatments for individuals with lupus".

Lady Gaga

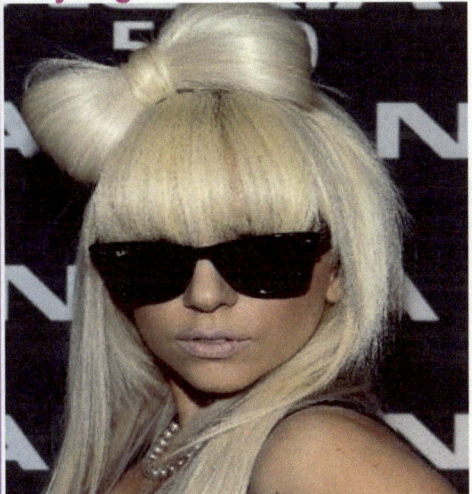

Lady Gaga's Aunt Joan died of lupus complications. In an interview for the Times she was asked if she had been tested for lupus and said: "Yes. but I don't want anyone to be worried." She did not actually reveal if the tests were negative or positive. She has since confirmed that her test shows she has 'borderline' lupus in an interview with Larry King 2nd June 2010.

Shannon Boxx

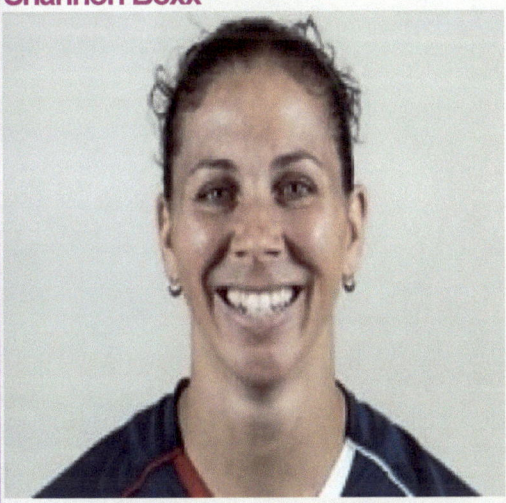

Shannon Boxx was diagnosed with lupus in 2007 when she was 30 years old. At the time, she was playing for the U.S. National Soccer Team and had begun feeling extremely fatigued; regular training sessions left her with joint pain and muscle soreness. She went public with her lupus diagnosis in April 2012 and is now working with the Lupus Foundation of America to create awareness about this chronic autoimmune disease that affects 1.5 million people in the U.S. Shannon took part in the London 2012 Olympic Games.

Michael Jackson

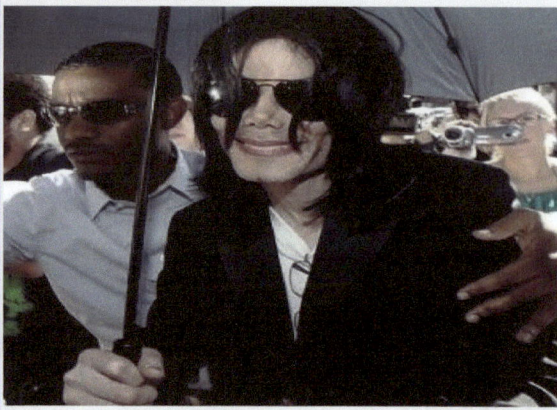

From CBS News" It reveals a rare court affidavit detailing several skin conditions that Jackson treats including Jackson's use of a powerful bleaching cream called Benoquin, because, according to his maid, "he does not like being black and he feels that blacks are not liked as much as people of other races." The affidavit also shows that Jackson was diagnosed with vitiligo and discoid lupus, which causes skin blotches".

Seal

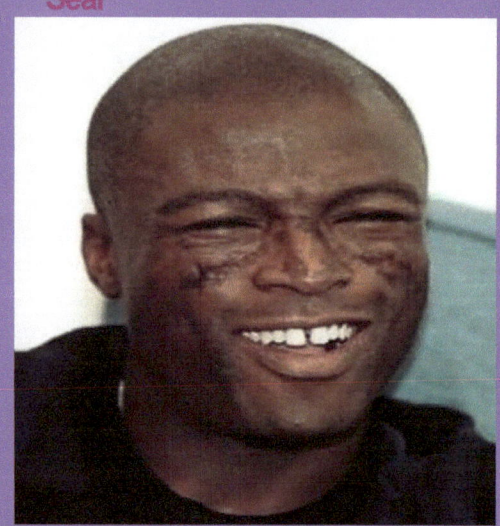

Questions about his facial scares persist. The scars were caused by a disease called lupus which Seal suffered from when he was a child. The strain of lupus **Seal** deals with causes blistering especially around the facial area, which when ruptured cause deep scarring. When questioned about his scares, Seal had often eluded to mystical or spiritual causes.

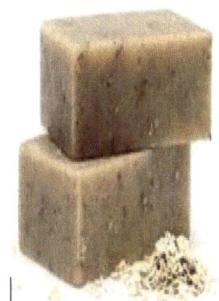

Oatmeal Turmeric Bar

4Oz

Product Line

Soaps 4oz

Bathe Soothers 8oz

Lotions 8oz

Butters 4oz

Products are made when ordered for the best result and a longer shelf life!

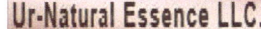

Ur-Natural Essence LLC.

Holistic & Therapeutic Products

Products that's Tailored for Natural Results

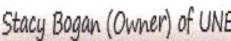

Stacy Bogan (Owner) of UNE

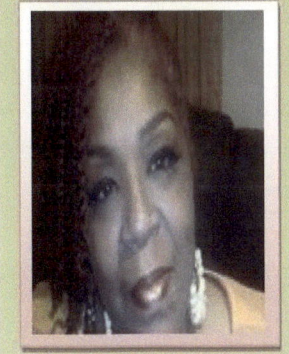

Tel: 770-895-6281

Ur-Natural Essence

UNe's products is a balance blends of essential oils and herbs for therapeutic purposes used in the morning and evening to help balance the bodies electrical energies, moisturize, restore, soothe aches and pain, and smooth skin's appearance.

UNe's Purpose

Our products purpose is to increase frequencies and enable the body heal itself by using natural product with no chemical, addictives, coloring, SLS or any animal by products that may clog your pores of cause any side effects.

Disclaimer

UNE is not claiming to heal any disease or medical problem but to assist with natural remedies seeing the results with proper use.

All our products are for external use only and if you are allergic to any of the essential oils (plants or herbs), Carrier oils (nuts or seeds) in our products please do not use. If pregnant or have HBP please consult with your physician before using any of UNE's products

What's in UNe's Products?

UNE ingredients are natural oils that are derived from plants, herbs and nuts for circulation, chronic pain and inflammation....... creating a soothing, restoring, rejuvenating and smoothing affect.

Who's UNe's dedicated Customer's?

Our Products are tailored for people with problematic skin.....our customers are people who have extremely dry, rashes, or any kind of outbreaks due to Lupus, Eczema, Diabetic, Dermatitis or Psoriasis.

Coconut Milk Butter Crème

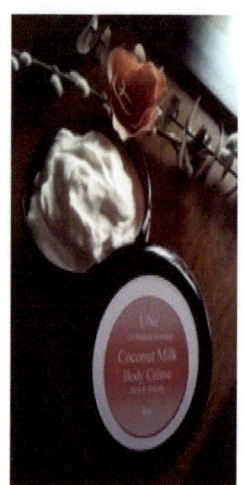

Moisturizing Butter Crème for normal to extremely dry Skin.

Ur-Natural Essence

Hiram, GA

30141

Phone: 770-895-6281

Email: naturalproduct31@gmail.com

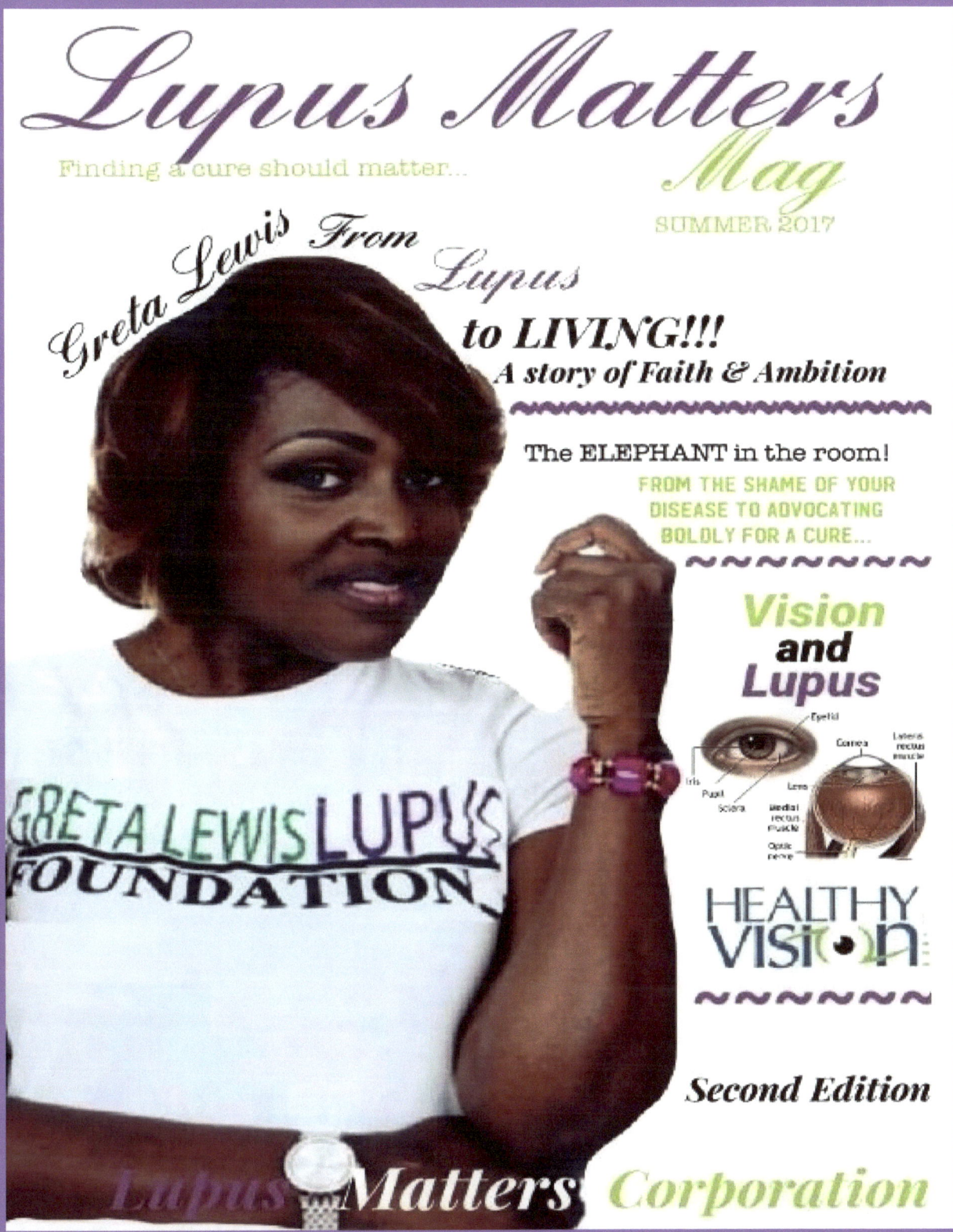

Advertising Prices

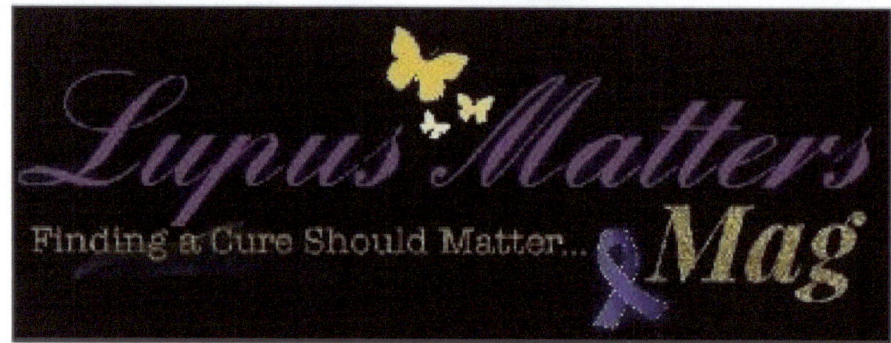

1/2 PAGE $50
FULL PAGE $75

We accept cash, debit & paypal

$40 **1/2 ONE HALF**	$20 1/4 PAGE	$20 1/4 PAGE
$40 **1/2 ONE HALF**	$20 1/4 PAGE	$20 1/4 PAGE

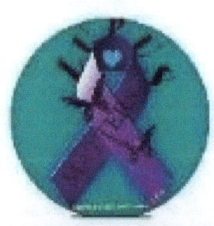

Lupus Matters Corporation

(404) 997-0761
LUPUSMATTERS@GMAIL.COM
www.lupusmatters.org

This magazine is published through the grace of God. Everything we do individually and as a company is to bring honor to HIS name.

Our magazine is to let Lupus warriors tell their story and how they are overcoming lupus.

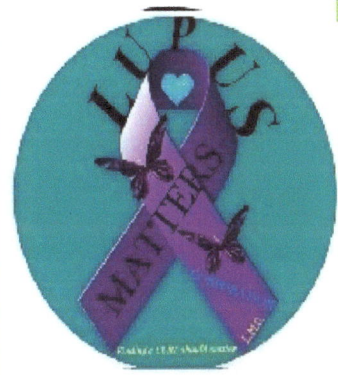

Thank you, for supporting our magazine

The ideas expressed by the writers are not necessarily that of the editor, the publisher or of Lupus Matters magazine.

The publisher reserves the right to reject any advertising or free submission or free submission at his discretion.

The publisher reserves the right to edit submission for space, grammar or to conform the content to fit the size of the magazine.

Founder & Publisher~
MONICA ELLIS
Associate Publisher~
JACQUELINE FOOTE

DOUGLASVILLE, GA.
30135
QUARTERLY CIRCULATION

dōTERRA

Wellness Advocate

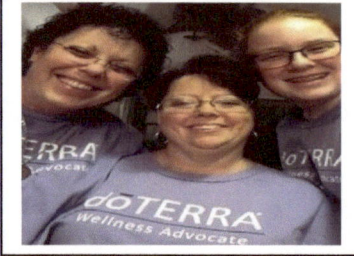

DōTERRA produces and distributes exceptionally high quality certified pure therapeutic grade essential oil's through more than 3 million independent distributors also known as Wellness Advocates around the world. Sherry Beckham and I are DōTERRA Wellness Advocates. Becoming DōTERRA Wellness Advocates is one of the BEST decisions we have made. "In addition to a premium line of essential oil's used by individuals and health-care professionals alike, the company also offers products that are naturally safe, purely effective, certified pure therapeutic grade essential oils, including personal care spa products, nutritional supplements, and healthy living products"(DōTERRA 2017). Since integrating a more natural holistic lifestyle our families are enjoying the benefits that essential oils have added to our health and well-being. "Essential oils can be used for a wide range of emotional and physical wellness applications. They can be used as single essential oils or in complex essential oil blends depending on user experience and desired benefit"(DōTERRA 2017).

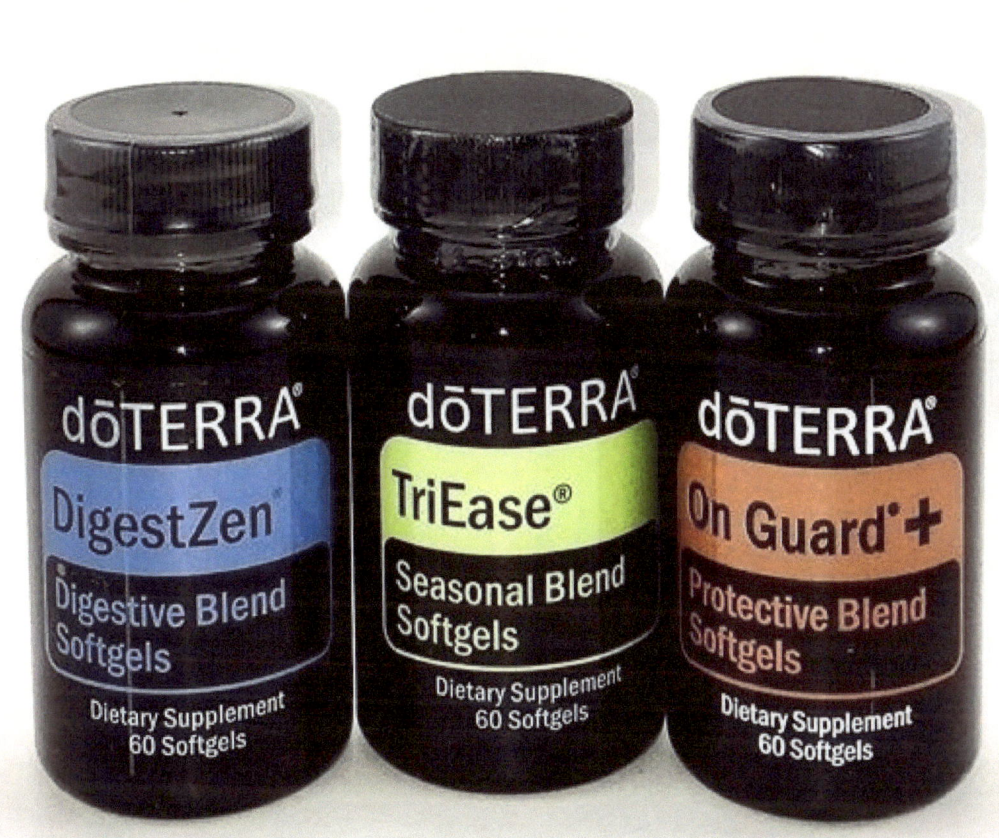

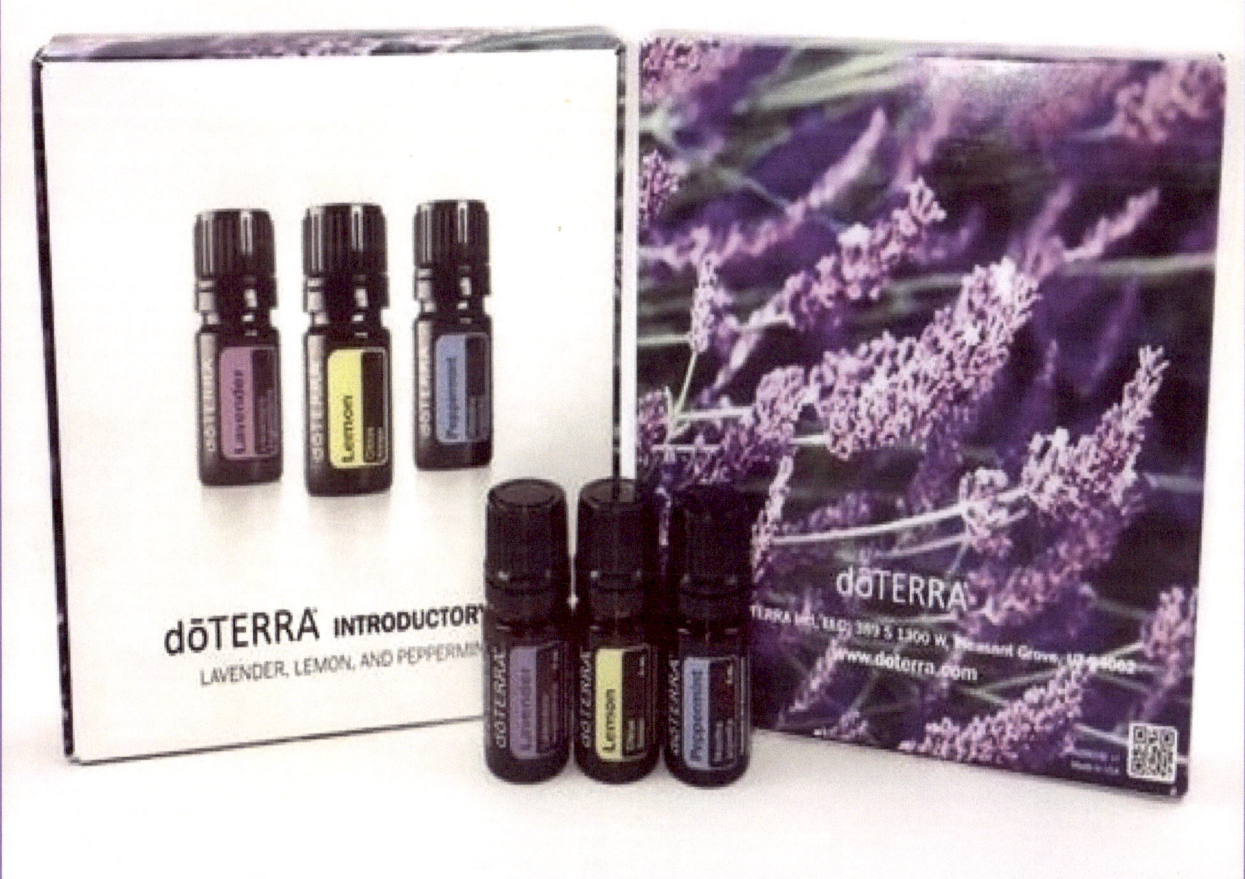

dōTERRA
deep
BLUE
RUB
dōTERRA
deep
BLUE
POLYPHENOL
COMPLEX™

dōTERRA
Geranium
AromaTouch
Lime
Elevation
dōTERRA
Tangerine
dōTERRA
Whisper

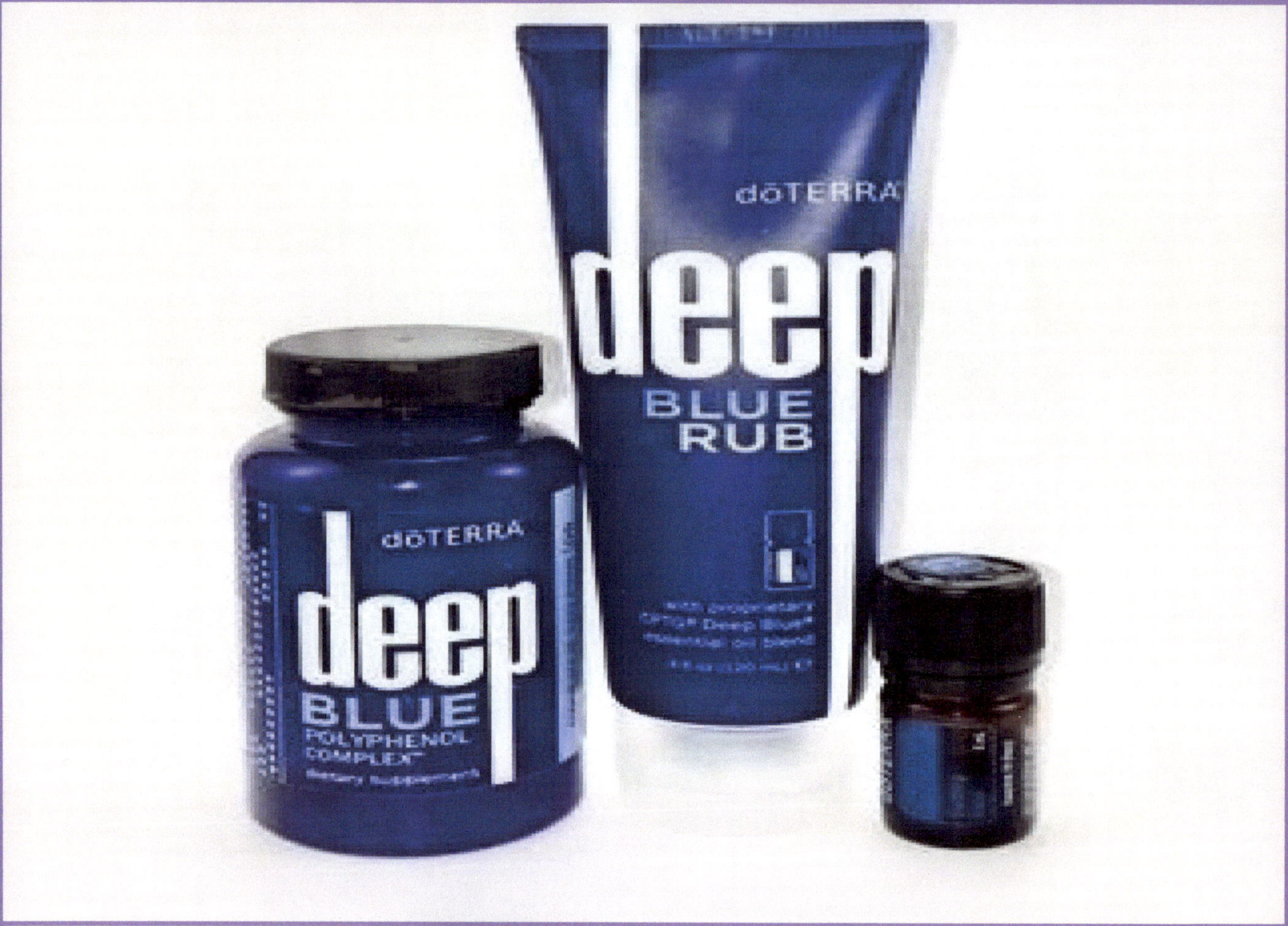

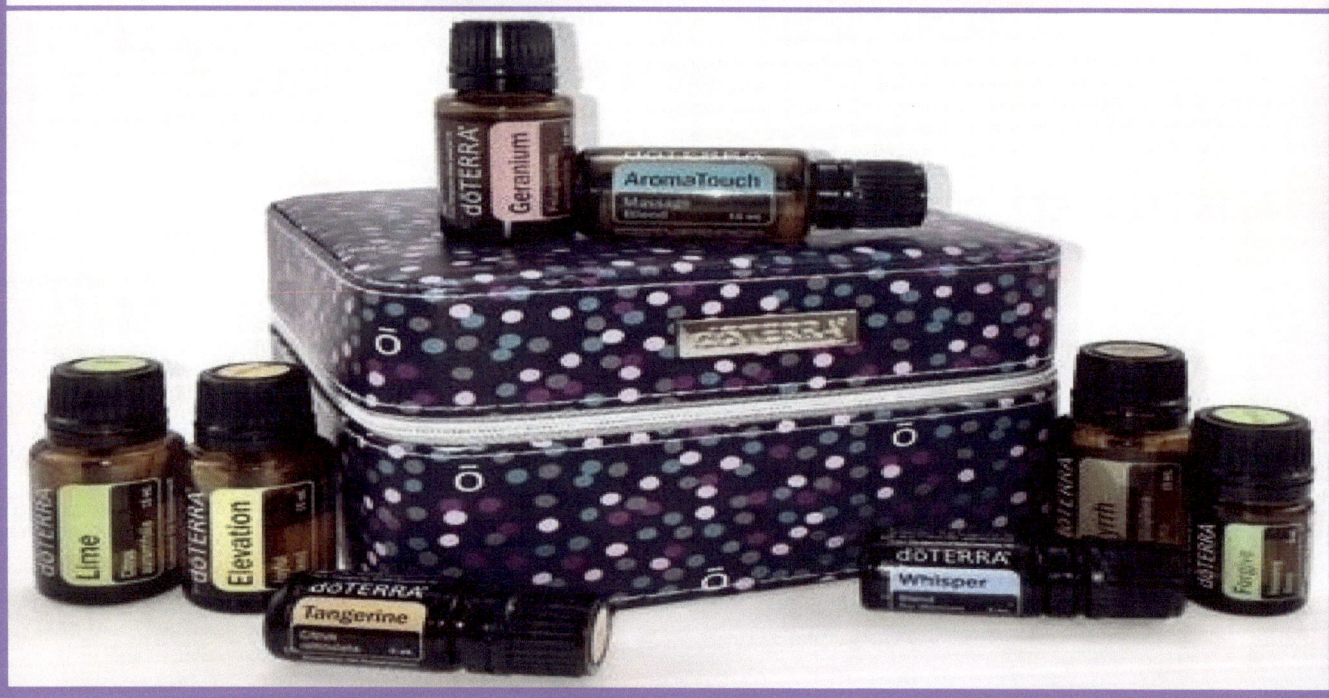

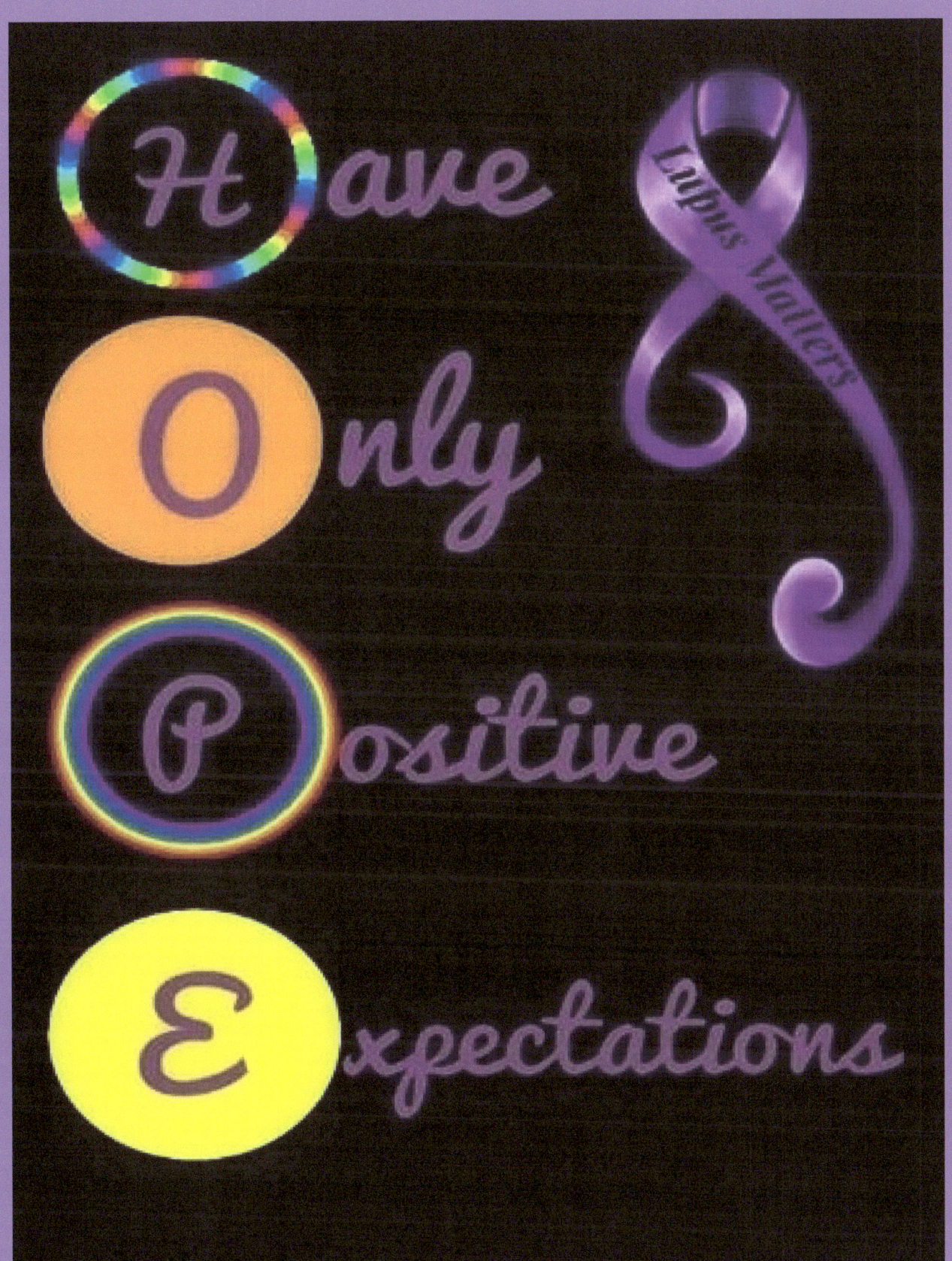

www.ingramcontent.com/pod-product-compliance
Lightning Source LLC
Chambersburg PA
CBHW041505280526
45792CB00004B/1139